HIV Education in Prisons

A Resource Book

Una Padel
Rose Twidale
John Porter

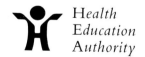

*Health
Education
Authority*

Health Education Authority
in association with SCODA

© Health Education Authority, 1992
Hamilton House, Mabledon Place, London WC1H 9TX

ISBN 1 85448 362 5

Designed by Cinamon and Kitzinger, London
Typeset by Type Generation Ltd, London
Printed by The KPC Group, London & Ashford, Kent

Contents

Foreword   v

Acknowledgements   vii

Introduction 1

1   HIV Education in Prisons   3

2   The Project   11

3   Organising Training   25

4   The Exercises   37

5   Other Initiatives in HIV and AIDS Education   79

6   Working Together – Prisons and the Community   97

Appendices

1   Examples of Training Needs Analyses   113

2   Handout on Training Methods
    by Jan Mojsa   115

3   Extracts from the Woolf Report   119

4   Useful Training Resources   127

5   Part 1: Directory of Prisons and Young Offender Institutions
    (YOIs), with corresponding District Health Authorities   129

    Part 2: Directory of Prisons/YOIs, with corresponding
    Prison Areas and Regional Health Authorities/Regional
    HIV Prevention Co-ordinators   147

6   Useful Organisations   153

7   Keeping up to Date   157

Glossary   161

Bibliography   165

Index   167

Foreword

The HIV/AIDS and Drug Misusing Offenders Project, funded by the Health Education Authority and based at the Standing Conference on Drug Abuse, has spent the past three years developing a model of HIV education for prisons. During this time the Project has gained considerable experience of negotiating with prison authorities, encouraging the setting up of multi-disciplinary HIV/AIDS committees in prisons and analysing training needs, as well as developing and running training programmes. It has also maintained contact with HIV education initiatives in prisons in other parts of the UK.

This resource book has been produced as a means of disseminating the work of the Project. It is intended both for people working in prisons as well as those in community-based agencies who wish to work with the prisons in their area. The work of the Project is described and details are given of the training programme developed. Other initiatives in the field are outlined and the experience of the Project staff in working with prisons provides the basis of a chapter designed to help prisons and community-based agencies work together. The book also contains lists of useful resources and addresses to facilitate contact between those working inside and out.

Acknowledgements

We would like to thank the Health Education Authority for providing the funding for the HIV/AIDS and Drug Misusing Offenders Project and the Standing Conference on Drug Abuse for hosting and managing it. The National AIDS Trust and the Inner London Probation Service continue to offer valuable guidance on the Project's Steering Committee. The Prison Department have been co-operative and supportive of the Project. Particular thanks are due to Len Curran and Peter Done of the Directorate of the Prison Medical Service for their help and support.

The prisons involved in the Project so far – Feltham, Pentonville and Belmarsh – provided the opportunities for the training methods to develop. We hope they feel they have gained from the process as well and would like to thank the management teams, training departments and other staff who have taken a particularly keen interest in our work and made contact with the prisons possible. The participants on the courses merit particular attention here. They enabled and assisted us in the development of our exercises, attended the courses with open minds, and are now facing the difficult task of continuing HIV education work in their prisons. Jan Mojsa, who worked with us on the Feltham training course, contributed a great deal to the shape of the course programme as it now stands. We thank her for all she did and for allowing us to reproduce her handout on training methods in Appendix 2. We have gained an enormous amount from contact with others involved in similar work throughout the country. We would particularly like to thank those who allowed their work to be featured in Chapter 5; John Pearce and Michael Clarke of Saughton Prison, Geoff Marlow of Bristol Prison, Robert Shepherd of Grendon Prison, Carey Godfrey of Suffolk Probation Service, Deborah Blackburn of Holloway Prison, Patricia McKenzie of First Community Health, Sue Whitlock of Leicestershire Probation Service and Di Robertson, the northern broker for HIV agencies and prisons.

This book would not have been possible without the help and support of Ruth Lowbury and Derek Bodell of the HEA, David Turner, Director, Hugh Dufficy, Deputy Director, and Kate Godwin, Publications Officer at SCODA. The hardest job of all – converting the handwritten scrawl into a neat typescript – was undertaken by Julie Howlin of SCODA with the assistance of Ann Defreitas, Barbara Gilbert and Ted Bentley. Particular thanks are due to them.

The Health Education Authority is grateful to the Controller of HM Stationery Office for permission to reproduce the two extracts in Appendix 3 from *Prison Disturbances April 1990: Report of an Inquiry by Lord Justice Woolf and Judge Stephen Tumim*, Cm 1456 (1991).

Introduction

Education is of crucial importance in halting the HIV pandemic. The task of providing HIV education on a routine basis to all prisoners is an enormous one. It is potentially very costly in terms of resources and, for many prisons, still appears to be of marginal relevance in comparison with more immediate concerns. Yet as the rate of HIV infection in the general population increases and more people start to develop symptoms, this state of affairs is likely to change.

This book offers practical strategies for providing HIV education in prisons. It is intended as a source of ideas and information to anyone intending to provide HIV education in prisons and as a resource for those already doing so. It is designed for people working in prisons and those employed in the health service and community-based drug and HIV agencies. A substantial part of the book consists of a detailed guide to the development of an integrated HIV training programme for prisons. This involves training a small group of uniformed staff in HIV awareness and enabling them to become HIV educators, running education sessions for prisoners or other prison staff. Every stage in the process is discussed and step-by-step instructions for the exercises used to train prison HIV educators are included. *Basic HIV information is not included.* An assumption is made that readers using these exercises will already have a good working knowledge and awareness of HIV. If this is not the case, extensive background reading (see Bibliography) or attendance at an HIV awareness course is recommended before attempting to embark on running any of the exercises described here. These exercises are designed to be run by two trainers working together and this may provide a useful opportunity for District HIV Prevention Co-ordinators or Health Promotion Officers to work directly with a member of the prison staff as co-trainer.

In addition this book offers an overview of other initiatives in the field and a guide for community-based agencies and prisons on working together. The appendices include a list matching prisons to their respective district health authorities with contact numbers for health authority HIV education workers, a directory of useful organisations and a guide to resources.

Scotland's prison system is administered separately from that of England and Wales. Unless otherwise stated all references to 'the prison system', 'the Prison Medical Service', etc. refer to the prison system in England and Wales since that is where the work of the Project was conducted.

Chapter 1

HIV Education in Prisons

The spread of HIV over the past decade has posed enormous medical, ethical and social problems for all areas of public health policy. Prisons inevitably share many of the problems experienced by other institutions; for example, hospitals and schools. These general issues, such as the provision of effective health education, confidentiality and maintaining the confidence of all staff in the information provided to them, carry their own particular difficulties in an overburdened prison system which has to balance many other priorities. Poor sanitation, chronic overcrowding and lack of employment for many prisoners all contribute to the tensions which occasionally manifest themselves in riots. More often the violence is turned inward. Fifty-six prisoners committed suicide in prison in England and Wales in 1990: against this background the problems of dealing with HIV and AIDS may appear less immediate. A total of seven prisoners died of AIDS-related diseases between 1985 and 1990. Yet there are distinct features which make the prison environment both unique and crucially important in the progression of the HIV pandemic. These features include:

• the high number of injecting drug users who pass through the prison system and are not in contact with helping agencies who could give HIV prevention information;

• a population, some of whom may be in monogamous relationships outside prison. They may find it difficult to negotiate safer sex on release, although either partner may have been involved in high-risk sex during the enforced separation;

• a predominantly young population, many of whom will embark on new sexual relationships soon after release, or possibly during their time in prison;

• people who have to cope with living with HIV or AIDS with little support from friends or relatives and less access to information than they could expect in the community;

- a population which is likely to contain a high number of 'rule breakers' who may be unlikely to think of the long-term consequences of their actions.

While good health and safety procedures should always be adopted, the poor standards of cleanliness and sanitation which exist in many prisons are not in themselves factors in the spread of HIV infection. The majority of prisoners are not sexually active in prison and do not inject drugs (Turnbull, Dolan and Stimson, 1991). However, for those who do, risks may be higher because condoms are not available for those wishing to have penetrative sex, and neither is clean injecting equipment or the most effective cleaning agent – bleach.

The Development of Prison Department Policy on HIV

Although the experience of the United States demonstrated in the early 1980s that HIV would become an issue for prisons, it was not until 1985 that the first prisoners with HIV were identified and recorded in England and Wales. Since then the numbers of HIV positive prisoners notified to the Prison Medical Service have been collected and give a cumulative total of 314 between March 1985 and August 1990 with the daily total generally between 50–65 over the past few years. These figures represent only prisoners who request or agree to an HIV antibody test and are found to be HIV positive, or those who choose to reveal to the prison medical authorities that they have HIV. Names and details of such prisoners are routinely passed to the Directorate of the Prison Medical Service by prison medical officers. The numbers obviously do not represent a complete picture of the extent of HIV infection in the prison population.

The point at which HIV was first identified in prisons was at a time when the media were often inaccurate and sensational in their reporting of HIV and AIDS. Industrial relations within the prison service were at a low ebb, with prison officers seeking to show that they were undervalued in order to preserve staffing levels and conditions of service which involved a large amount of overtime. The way in which HIV/AIDS policy developed seems to have been greatly affected by these circumstances. Outside observers find it difficult otherwise to understand why the Viral Infectivity Restrictions formulated in 1985 as a response to Hepatitis B should have been quite so precipitately applied to prisoners known to have HIV.

Viral Infectivity Restrictions (VIR) have effectively determined the conditions under which prisoners known to have HIV have been held. Initially those subject to VIR were detained in the hospital, unable to work or take part in sports. The restrictions were later modified to suggest that prisoners with HIV should be located on normal landings (though in single cells or sharing with others with the same diagnosis), could work but not with sharp objects and could be involved in sports other than contact sports. The modified regulations contained the caveat of isolation from the general population if the prisoner could not be trusted to act responsibly, or at the discretion of the medical officer. Although the HIV or AIDS diagnosis was supposed to remain confidential, the information that a prisoner was subject to VIR was available to anyone with an operational 'need to know'. Interpretations of the need to know varied greatly and it was never defined in policy.

Although the guidance on the location of prisoners known to have HIV changed, many prisons continued to keep those known to have the virus, or awaiting test results, in the prison hospital. Some prisons have even isolated prisoners judged to belong to a 'high-risk group', until they agreed to be tested and a negative test result was returned. Prison reform organisations assert that this coercive process was based on three false assumptions. First, the notion of a 'high-risk group', usually taken to mean gay men and injecting drug users, is very limited and ignores the risks taken by anyone involved in unprotected penetrative sex. Second, one negative test result has very limited validity because HIV antibodies may take three months to develop. Third, it implies, as does isolation of those known to have the virus, that HIV may be transmitted during the course of day-to-day prison life. This contradicts and undermines the messages conveyed by HIV education in prison.

At Wandsworth it was the doctor's refusal to use the hospital to house prisoners who were HIV positive and asymptomatic which resulted in the setting up of K1, a small unit used solely for people on VIR and isolated from the rest of Wandsworth's population. The extensive use of hospital accommodation for prisoners identified as having the virus and the development of K1 run counter to the spirit of national policy decisions, but for many prisons provide the easiest way out of a difficult situation. Where this has happened prison staff and prisoners alike seem to remain fearful of contact with those known to be infected and although many would acknowledge that there are likely to be unidentified prisoners and staff with HIV, they feel safer if those diagnosed are housed separately. The experience of HIV workers in prisons suggests that this in turn has resulted in an air of complacency in some prisons where health and safety practice is very poor. The use of Viral Infectivity Restrictions is currently under review by the Directorate of the Prison Medical Service. Such a review was also recommended by the report of the Woolf inquiry into prison disturbances (Woolf and Tumim, 1991).

Education

Widespread anxiety among prison staff about HIV and AIDS became particularly evident in 1986. At this time, according to the Department of Health, the Government was developing a strategy of HIV education designed for particular sections of the population. Providing education targeted specifically at prison staff was clearly a way of enabling them to feel more confident in dealing with HIV. To this end a committee was convened by the Directorate of the Prison Medical Service under the chairmanship of Len Curran, a principal psychologist in the prison service. Members of the committee were drawn both from within and outside the prison service, a welcome departure from practice hitherto. Representatives from Body Positive and the Terrence Higgins Trust, as well as outside medical experts, worked with prison service personnel on the production of a staff training package which became available in August 1987.

The package includes a video entitled *AIDS Inside* which provides information about HIV and AIDS as well as examining situations which may arise in prisons and which could create anxiety about HIV in staff. It was designed to be delivered by specially trained staff and the package also contains a manual outlining a step-by-step procedure for conducting the education session and for answering questions which may arise in discussion of the issues raised by the video.

Initially, this package was made available in all prisons, with targets for numbers to be trained set, although it appeared during the first year that the response was patchy. Now the training seems to occur mainly in the staff training college where all new prison officers receive a session on HIV as part of their training course.

Following the release of the staff training package, the AIDS Advisory Committee was reconvened, this time with representation from the

Department of Health, to create another aimed specifically at prisoners. Again the central component is a video entitled *AIDS Inside and Out* which graphically illustrates potential high-risk situations which may occur both in prison and after release. The difficulty that prisoners may have in believing information from the prison authorities is explicitly acknowledged as is the fact that unsafe sex, drug use and rape occur in prison.

The prisoner training package was sent to all establishments in March 1989 with instructions that every prisoner spending longer than four weeks in the prison system should be given the chance to see it. The reality is a little different. While some prisons have managed to incorporate the package into the prison routine through use on induction courses, pre-release or simply regular screenings of the video, others have found this difficult to achieve. A recent survey of 452 ex-prisoners (Turnbull, Dolan and Stimson, 1991) revealed that 58 per cent had not seen the video. The majority of these had not been offered the chance, but 30 had opted not to see it because of competing activities such as association (prisoners' recreation period) or paid work.

It is difficult to know why no use is being made of this valuable training resource at so many prisons. The fact that at those institutions where the package is in regular use a diversity of individuals and departments (including medical services, education, psychology, prison officers and outside agencies) take responsibility for it may offer some clue. In order that the localised needs of individual establishments be met, the Prison Medical Directorate did not offer any specific guidance on which department within each prison should undertake HIV education with prisoners.

Although many prisons seem to have been able to absorb this work, at others it appears to have become a political football with no one willing to take it on. At prisons with a high turnover of prisoners, fulfilling the prison department's own target constitutes a massive and continuing task. No additional resources were made available for this when the package was released. Current practice ranges from regular HIV education sessions accessible to all prisoners, to nothing at all in other institutions where the training package seems to have been consigned to the back of a dusty cupboard.

Since the production of *AIDS Inside and Out* the Prison Medical Directorate's training initiatives in this field have concentrated on specialised areas. Courses have been held for medical officers and nursing staff focusing on the care and support of people with HIV, with an emphasis on psychosocial needs. Prison Medical Service policy provides that all prisoners tested for HIV antibodies should receive pre- and post-test counselling. Unfortunately a shortage of trained counsellors has meant that this has not been achieved. A study by David Miller and Len Curran (1991) revealed that 27.8 per cent of the sample tested in prison had received pre-test counselling. Turnbull, Dolan and Stimson (1991) found that 55 per cent of those tested in prison from their sample were unaware of receiving any counselling. The Prison Medical Directorate is making efforts to ensure a rapid increase in the number of trained counsellors and the AIDS Advisory Committee has adapted the World Health Organisation preventive counselling module for use in prisons. The counselling course has been made available to prison staff from a range of disciplines. In addition a multi-disciplinary course for teams of five staff from each of six prisons has been piloted. This course allows participants the opportunity to consider what individual contribution they can make to the development of HIV policy as a member of a particular discipline or profession within the prison. Each multi-disciplinary team is then given time to devise an HIV/AIDS strategy appropriate to the prison from which they have come and is required to set targets to achieve six and twelve months from the course.

This multi-disciplinary course is clearly designed to promote the development of good and coherent practice at the level of the individual institution. At some it will undoubtedly raise the issues of HIV and AIDS again after a period during which they have been ignored. However, it will take a considerable time to provide sufficient courses to enable representatives from all prisons to attend.

The Terrence Higgins Trust has recently produced an educational booklet for prisoners about HIV and AIDS (*HIV and AIDS: a Booklet for Prisoners*, 1991) and the Prison Department have undertaken to distribute it to all prisoners.

Local Action

There is no reason for individual prisons to wait until an opportunity to attend the multi-disciplinary course is offered before attempting to address the issues of HIV and AIDS. A number of localised initiatives are already under way and some of them are described in Chapter 5. Initial stage in taking the issue further might include:

● convening a multi-disciplinary HIV/AIDS committee to oversee policy and development of work in this area;
● conducting a review of HIV/AIDS policy within the prison with particular regard to confidentiality. It might be useful to produce a local HIV/AIDS policy document;
● assessing the extent and effectiveness of current HIV education for prisoners and staff;
● conducting a review of local health and safety policy and practice and providing additional training if necessary;
● ensuring that pre- and post-test counselling is available to any prisoner requesting a blood test for HIV antibodies and that this is provided by someone specifically trained in pre- and post-test counselling;
● enabling prisoners to have easy access to suitably trained staff or workers from outside agencies who can provide support and advice to those concerned about HIV and AIDS;
● making contact with the local District HIV Prevention Co-ordinator to explore what assistance can be provided in the development of HIV education and counselling.

In spite of the competing priorities faced by any prison it is vital that all staff and prisoners are provided with enough information to enable them to keep themselves and others safe from HIV, that expert counselling is available to those who choose to have an HIV antibody test, and that well-informed advice and support is available to anyone with concerns in this area.

Chapter 2

The Project

The HIV/AIDS and Drug Misusing Offenders Project is a collaborative venture funded by the Health Education Authority and located at the Standing Conference on Drug Abuse. The National AIDS Trust and Inner London Probation Service are also represented on the Steering Committee. The rationale for the original Project proposal was derived from the Advisory Council on the Misuse of Drugs (ACMD) report *AIDS and Drug Misuse*, Part I (1988). The report noted that there was a particular proportion of the drug using population for whom current service provision appeared inadequate – those who after offending are received into custody or sent to a bail or probation hostel. The Project consists of two distinct elements: one involving prisons and the other probation and bail hostels. The latter is not described in this book.

Aims and Objectives

The Prison Project aims to create a method of providing information and education about HIV and AIDS to people living and working in prisons. While the underlying rationale centres on the particular needs of those drug users who may not be in contact with services and therefore have no access to HIV information, any educational effort must be available to all. Many drug users do not reveal their drug use to the medical officer when they enter prison, and a high proportion do not have convictions for drug offences. It would be futile to attempt to provide such information only to drug users, since those not identified may be putting themselves at greatest risk. In any event the provision of HIV education to all prisoners is important because some may be engaged in high-risk sexual activity. Not only may prison staff also be involved in high-risk activity in their personal lives but in the prison both staff and prisoners may be subjecting people known or believed to have HIV to unnecessary prejudice and privation because they are simply unaware of the facts.

The Project was originally to employ two people for a minimum of two years. As it evolved, an extension for one more year and additional funds to employ another project worker in the third year were made available by the Health Education Authority.

Soon after the beginning of the Project the original proposal was submitted to the Directorate of the Prison Medical Service (DPMS) for approval. Some clarification was required on a few points, and a revised proposal for prison work was approved in January 1990.

The agreed objectives were:

1. To assess those staff training needs not met by current Prison Department training initiatives in the fields of drug use and HIV/AIDS issues.
2. To provide any additional training or information necessary for staff about drug use and HIV/AIDS.
3. To assess those prisoner education needs not met by current Prison Department training initiatives in the fields of drug use and HIV/AIDS issues.
4. To assist staff to provide additional health education to prisoners resulting from this assessment.
5. To develop links between each prison and appropriate community-based organisations which may be able to develop further the educational work initiated by the Project after the end of its lifespan.
6. To develop appropriate support networks (where these do not already exist) for staff working in HIV/AIDS and drug education, and caring for prisoners with HIV disease.

In order to develop a method of achieving these objectives which would be relevant to different situations, it was agreed that the Project should approach Feltham Young Offenders Institution (remand and convicted young males), Pentonville (remand and convicted adult males) and Cookham Wood (convicted adult females). Work undertaken at Feltham YOI and Pentonville is described below. Fortunately for Cookham Wood, but not for the Project, a programme of HIV education was already under way when the Project's initial approach was made. The same was true of Bullwood Hall women's prison. It now appears that the Project may be able to undertake some work at Holloway Prison, but at the time of writing (August 1991) this is still under negotiation.

Sadly, this means that the Project work described here does not take account of the particular needs of women prisoners. A description of work already being undertaken by a prison officer at Holloway is included in Chapter 5. Some of the training methods developed by the Project would, in all probability, be equally appropriate for use with women as with men, but it is important that the specific training needs present within a women's prison are adequately assessed. The suitability of specific exercises could then be gauged and new elements introduced where appropriate.

Since the response from Cookham Wood and Bullwood Hall left the Project with only two prisons to work with, we made an approach to Belmarsh Prison just before it opened in April 1991. As well as providing a third prison with which to work, Belmarsh offered the opportunity to develop the Project model in a new prison, creating an interesting contrast with Pentonville. This offer was accepted and training undertaken at Belmarsh is also described.

As the Project developed, a potential conflict between the objectives agreed with the Prison Department and the need to operate as a demonstration project emerged. The objectives suggested provision of a continuing service to the prisons concerned in terms of supplementing existing HIV education initiatives. However, the Project was short term and intended to create a method of working which might be replicated elsewhere. This last aspect meant that the method designed should not be too labour intensive since most community-based agencies do not enjoy the luxury of two or three workers who can be deployed on prison work full time.

Development of a Training Model

After learning about the training models already under development at Saughton and Bristol Prisons (see Chapter 5 for further information) we decided to adopt a similar approach. This involves training a small group of staff to undertake the training of other staff and inmates. While demanding a high degree of input from Project workers in the short term, it sets in motion a means of providing HIV and AIDS information and in the long run the group of trained staff should be able to support one another. They should be able to gain updated information on HIV and AIDS from community-based organisations they have been put in touch with by the Project.

The next question to emerge was where to draw the nucleus of staff to be trained as HIV educators from. Our individual experiences with many prisons informed our decision to offer training exclusively to uniformed staff. The reasons for this were numerous. Prison officer trainers are more likely to enjoy greater credibility with their uniformed colleagues, who may be suspicious of the motives behind HIV education, than members of other professional disciplines within the prison. Prisoners also have more contact with prison officers than with any other group of prison staff and this high level of contact may mean that prisoners are afforded greater opportunities to ask questions informally of the officer/educators following training sessions than they would if HIV educators were drawn from other disciplines. We feared that probation officers, teachers, psychologists, etc. would be unlikely to be able to make a long-term commitment to the provision of HIV education. There seems to be a trend towards prison officers becoming increasingly involved in running induction and pre-release courses and developing their roles as personal officers. HIV education fits neatly into the idea of developing the professional role of the prison officer advocated by many within the Prison Department, the Woolf Report and the Prison Officers Association.

A further reason for making the training available exclusively to uniformed staff was that we felt it would be important for the trained group to develop a clear identity and to nominate a co-ordinator from within. Although we had no specific evidence to support us, we felt that the involvement of a probation officer or teacher, for example, might result in the officer/educator group being led or co-ordinated by someone not so directly involved in the education work. This would dilute the strong sense of ownership and control over the education package that we try to foster within the officer/educator group.

This method of training a small nucleus of prison staff to educate others has developed in the three prisons in which the Project has been operational to date. The main problem it presents is that it demands a high level of commitment to HIV education from the prison's management team. The reduction in prison officers' working hours, as the final stages of the Fresh Start agreement are implemented, means that many prisons face staffing problems. Unless there is a lasting agreement that HIV education is of sufficiently high priority to merit the release of staff from normal duties on a regular basis, this model of training is likely to run into difficulties. However, it is difficult to devise any other means of HIV education provision which could be made available to all staff and prisoners that would make less demand on resources.

Inevitably, members of the core group of officer/educators are likely to move to other prisons or take on more responsibilities which mean leaving the HIV training group. If the officer/educators are able to meet together regularly and develop a strong group identity it should be possible for further staff to be recruited and trained by the group with input from outside agencies. Once again the overt support of the prison is essential to this process.

Accounts of work conducted at Feltham, Pentonville and Belmarsh follow and then further discussion of some of the key elements and decisions taken during the development of the Project.

Feltham Young Offenders Institution and Remand Centre

Feltham has a population of approximately 750 young male prisoners, 500 of whom are in the remand centre. It is one of the largest young offender institutions in Europe.

Initial contact with Feltham was made with the Governor. The Project was then invited to attend a senior management policy meeting in order to introduce the Project and discuss ideas about how we might work within the prison.

Arrangements were made for us to carry out a training needs analysis on a sample of 22 staff from different grades, locations and departments within the institution. The psychology department was instrumental in organising the practical details of this exercise. We interviewed staff for 30–45 minutes, using a schedule to guide our questions which were designed to determine levels of knowledge, concerns about HIV at work, and what kind of training or information staff had already received about HIV and AIDS.

While there was a range of responses a few features stood out. Almost all staff interviewed recognised that, although prisoners known by the Prison Medical Officer to have HIV were located in the prison hospital, all staff were likely to be working with other prisoners who have the virus and are unaware of it, or choose not to disclose the fact, on the units. All staff were aware of the main routes of transmission, but a number were unsure about whether there was a risk associated with contact with saliva or urine. Most felt that they were not at risk in the work setting, though many expressed the view that others felt differently. A majority felt that they would benefit from HIV/AIDS updates and there was dissatisfaction with the level of information currently available.

We used the information gathered to formulate a proposal for staff training at Feltham. We suggested training a group of officers in HIV/AIDS awareness and basic education skills, who would then use the training sessions to design and present a training package suitable for use with other staff and ultimately prisoners. We proposed working with four officers on four days staggered over a month and a half, in order to allow people to assimilate information and also not to be too disruptive to the shift system. In addition to the training, we also recommended that a multi-disciplinary HIV/AIDS steering committee be convened to support and monitor the progress of the training group and take into account health and safety and policy issues that might arise.

A further five months elapsed before the training took place. During this time volunteer officers were selected, contact was made with the training department to see if we could use the facilities, an appropriate course was designed and an HIV/AIDS steering committee was established as we had recommended. Membership of the committee included the Head of Custody, the Senior Probation Officer, the Senior Psychologist, an education officer, a senior hospital officer, a training officer and a Prison Officers Association representative.

The course was run by a project worker and Jan Mojsa, a trainer who had been involved in developing the health education pack *Learning About AIDS*. Geoff Marlow, HIV Education Officer from Bristol Prison also ran a session on one of the days.

The course was well received by participants who enthusiastically designed and practised a two-hour package of basic information and then negotiated with the prison for two further days to refine the package. The course for staff is now offered as part of the monthly staff training programme, and all staff are ultimately expected to attend.

The training group have elected a co-ordinator. They have adapted the package for use with prisoners and are in the process of trying to ensure that every remand prisoner who is in Feltham for the first time receives the basic information. Steps are in hand to do the same for the convicted population. The Parole Release Scheme, a drugs agency providing services to prisoners in south-east England, is also involved in running some of the sessions with prisoners.

Although Feltham is currently endeavouring to ensure that both staff and prisoner education sessions are run on a consistent basis, both the officer/educators and their managers share the difficulty of making sufficient time for this to happen. If the officers are running HIV education they are not available for their normal duties, but their managers are not provided with other staff to cover for them.

The trained staff are now included in the membership of the steering committee which has broadened its brief to include issues concerning the provision of advice to individuals and pre- and post-test counselling. As well as having a psychologist and a probation officer trained in counselling, some of the officers have attended the south-west prison area training course in basic counselling skills. With the committee and the medical department they are looking at how a confidential service can be established in Feltham.

Further information is available from Senior Officer Chris Denning, HIV/AIDS Co-ordinator, Feltham YOI, Bedfont Road, Feltham, Middlesex TW13 4ND. Tel: 081-890 0061.

Pentonville Prison

Pentonville is a large adult male prison located in central London with about a third of the population on remand.

Contact with Pentonville was first made with the Governor to introduce the project. Arrangements were made through the head of inmate activities to meet with staff from the hospital, education, pre-release and induction, training and probation departments. The intention of this was to build up a picture of the type of work that had been carried out on HIV and AIDS issues and to look at what could realistically be developed within the prison. A report based on this reconnaissance was then presented to a multi-disciplinary group of staff interested in the issues raised by HIV, AIDS and drugs. This group included representatives from the hospital, probation, pre-release and community agencies already working in the prison, an officer and the head of inmate activities.

While the need for staff to receive accurate information was recognised, it was decided that the initial priority was to provide basic HIV health education for prisoners, as it was clear from contact with all departments that most prisoners were not receiving HIV information. At that stage the pre-release and induction training staff were, and still are, providing sessions on drug use and HIV, run by the Parole Release Scheme (a drugs agency providing a service specifically to prisoners in south-east England) and an HIV advice worker from the local district health authority. However, only small numbers of prisoners are able to attend these courses because they are only open to convicted prisoners and places are limited. Similarly, the education department incorporated an HIV component within a general health course. It was decided that the prison would aim at ensuring greater coverage within the prisoner population of *AIDS Inside and Out* together with a discussion of its implications. In order to do this more staff would need to be trained in HIV and AIDS awareness and in running a focused education group.

The multi-disciplinary group decided to continue meeting in order to look at the many logistical problems that would need to be overcome if this aim was to be met and to co-ordinate initiatives around HIV and also drugs.

The Project undertook to provide basic staff training on HIV and AIDS and to enable a training package for prisoners to be developed. An officer, who has now been made HIV/AIDS Co-ordinator, undertook the recruitment of a group interested in carrying out this work with the help of the training department. Negotiation was also carried out with the training department to agree appropriate dates and the use of the training facilities and equipment.

In May 1991 eight people attended the four-day course. The course had developed from the one used at Feltham but the content included more information and looked in greater detail at safer sex and safer drug use. The overall aims remained the same. Another change was to arrange the course in a four-day consecutive block rather than as a total of four days spread over six weeks.

The course was enthusiastically received. Participants were able to devise an education package which they felt would be both useful and interesting to prisoners. Since the course, the group have negotiated a further day to refine their presentations and now have a representative on the multi-disciplinary group.

Further information is available from Bill Moss, HIV/AIDS Co-ordinator, HM Prison Pentonville, Caledonian Road, London N7 8TT. Tel: 071-607 5353.

Belmarsh Prison

Belmarsh is a large, new prison for adult men in south-east London. It is a category B prison and holds both remand and convicted prisoners.

The nature of the contact with Belmarsh has differed in a number of ways from that with Feltham and Pentonville. One of the main differences is that the Project approached the prison with a 'ready made' training package, thereby cutting down the negotiating period considerably.

Initial contact was made with the Governor who referred the Project to the prison's medical service. The health care centre had already written an HIV/AIDS policy which does not involve the adoption of Viral Infectivity Restrictions. It aims to preserve medical confidentiality and advocates the adoption of a health and safety policy that treats all body fluid spillages as if they could contain the virus.

A meeting with the health care managers established that the prison was very interested in the idea of a group of staff being trained to offer basic HIV education to other staff and to prisoners. The next step was to organise a seminar for middle management to introduce the Project, discuss the aims of the training and to elicit their support. This was felt to be especially important as involving prison and hospital officers in HIV education inevitably involves some release from their other duties.

The course was organised through the staff training department. An advertisement was prepared and made available to staff on each unit and was aimed at basic grade hospital or discipline officers. The training department dealt with recruitment for the course and arranged for participants to attend in civilian dress.

The course was well received and was attended by 12 staff. The feedback from participants indicated a high level of interest in the idea of being involved in the basic education process. While the prison was initially reluctant to set up an HIV steering committee, moves are now afoot to establish such a group to provide management support and to enable prisoner training to be undertaken.

Further information is available from Peter Bremner, Hospital Officer, HM Prison Belmarsh, Western Way, Thamesmead, Woolwich, London SE28 OEB. Tel: 081-317 2436.

Summary

The general process adopted by the Project can be summarised as follows:

Letter to Governor outlining Project

↓

Meeting with Governor, head of inmate activities, head of training, etc. to outline proposed work. It is helpful to meet as many of the prison management team as possible in a single meeting

↓

Conduct training needs analysis among cross section of staff

↓

Report to policy committee with written proposal for training and clear indication of staff time required and suggest setting up of multi-disciplinary HIV committee

↓

Advertise for prison officer volunteers for training

↓

Four-day training course for 8–16 officers including development of a specific package for the individual prison   →   HIV committee receives feedback on the progress of the training package and reports to the policy committee

↓   ↓

Trained officers spend extra time practising the package   ←   HIV committee ensures that trained staff are released from normal duties to attend practice sessions, training and monthly meeting for trainers

↓

Education sessions for staff and/or prisoners start

It is difficult to provide any reliable indication of how long this process may take. The Project's experience suggests between six and ten months is a likely time-scale from start to finish. Arranging to conduct a training needs analysis, doing so and reporting back to the policy committee may take at least a month. Training courses usually have to be arranged with the training department five to eight weeks before they take place. Because of staff leave it is difficult to achieve much during the school summer holidays or over the Christmas period which adds to delays.

Initial Contact

The Project made initial contact with the governor of each prison enabling him to decide how best to deal with our proposal. One governor met us with his senior staff to find out more, one passed our letter to the head of inmate activities and the third to the health care service within the prison. The other two governors declined the offer of our HIV training model since HIV education was already established in their prisons.

Many community-based organisations make their initial approach via the probation, education or psychology departments. This can sometimes be a very effective way of gaining access to a prison and of forging an alliance which can lead to productive co-operative work.

This Project decided not to approach the prisons in that way because we wanted to create the broadest possible base for our work. While the foothold afforded by going in through a particular department can be beneficial, it can also be detrimental if that department does not enjoy good relationships with other departments in the prison. In some prisons we also sensed a reluctance on the part of some departments to become too closely associated with the HIV education issue. Realising what a gigantic task it would be, they were fearful of being swamped by it and achieving nothing else. Once established within the prisons we were pleased to work closely with people from a number of departments, but we felt it essential to be, and appear to be, as independent as possible in the early stages.

Another advantage of writing to the governor initially is that, even though it is likely that the letter will be passed on, the approval of the governor is very important in the long term. Prison governors have a range of priorities for the allocation of staff, and they are expected to report on the progress made in HIV education in their annual reports. With so many priorities a direct approach may not ensure success, but it may be perceived as both courteous and helpful.

Training Needs Analysis

Before any training was carried out it was essential to determine both the level of existing knowledge and also the attitude of staff towards HIV and AIDS and HIV training. To do this, structured interviews were conducted with a sample of staff from all grades at Feltham, the first prison we worked with as described above. While it may not be essential to conduct such a formal training needs analysis at each prison, it has been very important to spend some time talking to members of different departments each time. This affords an opportunity not only to judge levels of HIV awareness and local attitudes, but also to get a sense of the way in which each prison operates. This can be important when it comes to suggesting ways in which HIV education can be carried forward in that prison. Examples of the training needs analysis used by the project can be found in Appendix 1.

Multi-disciplinary HIV/AIDS Committees

At every prison the Project has worked with we have encouraged the establishment of a multi-disciplinary HIV/AIDS committee. This approach is in line with current Prison Department policy which encourages the adoption of a multi-disciplinary approach. There are a number of advantages to be gained from it. HIV and AIDS raise many issues affecting a wide range of staff in prisons and a committee enables local policy decisions to be made and national policy to be implemented in a coherent and consistent manner. It provides a forum to enable discussion to take place and ensures that, while different departments are not involved in unnecessary duplication of effort, no gaps in provision emerge unnoticed. In terms of HIV education, using the model developed by this Project, such a committee has a role in ensuring that the officer/educators are able to use their skills in training staff or prisoners. This is likely to involve intervening with managers to release staff to run education sessions or to meet regularly with their fellow trainers. The committee can also provide an avenue through which the officer/educator group can communicate with senior management if necessary.

Membership of the committee should be determined according to the local situation (for example, HIV counselling is provided by various departments in different prisons). Generally, it is useful to include the head of inmate activities, a representative of the medical services, a member of the training department, a probation officer, a psychologist, a teacher and at least one member of the officer/educator group. Some prisons also find it useful to involve representatives from community-based HIV/AIDS organisations and from unions representing prison staff. The local District HIV Prevention Co-ordinator may also be able to make a valuable contribution facilitating access to other community-based services.

HIV Education Packages

An important and distinctive aspect of the Project's 'training for officer/educators' course is the opportunity afforded to participants to design an HIV education package for themselves. The alternative would have been for us to create a prison education package and simply train the officers to run it on the final day of our course. We prefer to encourage participants to design their own because it is then tailored to suit the exact climate in which it will be delivered. The officer/educators are far more likely to be able to judge how particular exercises will be received by either staff or inmates at their prison than we are. It is also essential that they should feel comfortable running the package. When officer/educators have created their own package they inevitably have a considerable personal investment in making it work and in ensuring that it is used. Another benefit is that if for some reason there is a need to change the structure or contents of the package at some time in the future, the officer/educators are familiar with the processes involved in formulating a training package and are likely to be able to modify it as required. We have encouraged each group to include the video *AIDS Inside and Out* as an integral part of the package. It affords a good factual account of HIV and AIDS which would otherwise be a particularly difficult task for the officer/educators to carry out consistently. Use of the video enables the officer/educators to concentrate on attitudes to HIV and on persuading the prisoners or staff they are working with to consider what changes are necessary to their own behaviour.

Chapter 3

Organising Training

Introduction

No matter how good the training course that may eventually be offered within a prison, its ultimate success or failure may rest on the preparation and negotiation that precede it and the support it receives afterwards. This chapter describes the aims and objectives of the training offered and some of the processes the Project developed to set up, evaluate and maintain training in prisons. It is intended as a guide which may be useful to those wishing to set up similar training in a prison for the first time, as well as a potential source of ideas for people already working in prisons.

Aims and Objectives

Clear aims and objectives are very important. Little training is currently offered within prison establishments on HIV and AIDS and related issues, which can make it difficult to get the balance right between attempting to meet actual training need and developing a realistic course curriculum. Our aims and objectives were as follows.

The overall aim of the course is to enable volunteer prison officers to develop their own HIV education package for either staff or prisoners. The course serves as an introduction to some of the key issues relating to HIV and AIDS. It does not attempt to turn prison officers into full-time trainers but introduces them to the process of HIV health education and then looks at ways they can develop their skills and knowledge in the context of their job.

The objectives of the course are:

● to provide up-to-date information about HIV, AIDS, safer sex and safer drug use;

- to examine attitudes to HIV and AIDS, to people with the virus, sexuality, safer sex and drug use;
- to demonstrate different techniques of providing training and information.

It seeks to achieve this by providing the opportunity:

- to enable participants to develop a two-hour education package on HIV for staff or prisoners at the prison concerned;
- to practise delivery of part of this package.

The course developed by the Project adopts a participative learning approach. It aims to build on participants' existing knowledge, take them through the process of developing a short educational session, and increase their confidence and knowledge in discussing HIV and AIDS. Many of the exercises involve small group, individual or pair work. They aim to encourage participants to work together to share concerns and anxieties as well as knowledge and understanding.

The course is designed for prison officers and hospital officers and takes place over four days. A four-day block often seems to be the easiest format to arrange with the prison training department and it allows participants to concentrate on the issues and develop as a group. Since the intention is that they eventually become the prison HIV educators and work in pairs, it is important that they are able to get to know other group members.

The training group should be kept small. Between 8 and 16 seems a reasonable size to tackle some of the more sensitive issues within the programme.

Course Trainers

Trainers may come from within the prison or from a health education or care agency in the HIV or drugs field. A training team of staff from inside and outside prison may be the best way to combine both an in-depth knowledge of prison working and community-based facilities with expertise in HIV/AIDS and risk reduction. More important, the training team needs to feel confident in the following:

- basic knowledge of HIV and AIDS;
- understanding of discrimination faced by groups and individuals because of HIV;

- knowledge of risk reduction strategies;
- ability to facilitate discussions that will include attitudes to sex, drug use, sexuality and race;
- preparedness to work within prisons and with prison officers.

It can be effective for two trainers to work together in terms of sharing workload, expertise and responsibility for assessing how things are going and whether any adjustments need to be made to the way exercises are conducted. However, if two trainers who have not worked together before are planning to run an HIV course it is essential that sufficient preparation time is built in. This allows not only discussion as to who is leading which parts of the programme and how, but also what language is to be used when discussing HIV and AIDS, sex, drug use, sexuality and race. There are many areas of uncertainty and it is essential that co-trainers have decided in advance how they will tackle these areas. Consistency between the two trainers or at least awareness of, and ability to explain, any differences in attitude are essential to the credibility of the training. One way of exploring whether any important differences do exist might be for the trainers to do the attitude statement exercise (Chapter 4) in private while planning the training.

Pre-course Planning

During negotiations with management (described in Chapter 2) the history and current state of HIV and AIDS initiatives in the prison may become clear. However, before finalising the content of the course it is useful to obtain a more complete picture of the prison's response to HIV and AIDS. This can help in addressing specific concerns that may be peculiar to that establishment and can indicate how the issues might be addressed in the future. There are several ways such an exercise can be undertaken. Short, confidential interviews can be useful in establishing an idea of levels of knowledge and current concerns about HIV and AIDS and also current policy, practice and training programmes within the prison. A semi-structured interview, or even a more formal training needs analysis similar to those used by the Project, may help. Examples of the interview schedules used at Feltham and Pentonville can be found in Appendix 1. Visits to different locations in the prison can be arranged with management in order to talk to staff on duty that day, or the officers who are to be trained can be interviewed if they have already been recruited (see 'Negotiation with the Staff Training Department' below). This process can be time-consuming, so it is useful to include details of an intention to do this during initial negotiation. The final content and structure of the programme will thus be informed by the course aims and objectives, information from the prison about needs, and the views and strengths of the trainers.

It is essential to draw up a detailed schedule of the exercises that will take place each day. The final programme for a four-day course may be similar to the programme which was used at Pentonville and Belmarsh:

Example of a Course Programme

Day One

  9.30 Introduction to the course
  9.45 Ground rules
10.15 Facts about HIV and AIDS
10.45 Coffee
11.00 Sorting the facts from the myths
12.30 Lunch
  1.30 Moral dilemmas role play
  3.00 Tea
  3.15 Attitude statement exercise
  4.15 Closing exercise
  4.30 Close

Day Two

  9.30 Opening exercise
10.00 HIV, AIDS and prisons, including showing of video *AIDS Inside and Out*
11.00 Prison situation exercise
12.30 Lunch
  1.30 Drug use and HIV
  2.45 Tea
  3.00 Safer sex
  4.15 Closing exercise
  4.30 Close

Day Three
  9.30 Opening exercise
  9.45 Discussion of training methods
 10.30 Discussion on devising an educational package
 11.30 Coffee
 11.45 Devising an educational package continued
 12.30 Lunch
  1.30 Devising an educational package continued
  2.00 Pair work on educational package
  3.00 Tea
  3.15 Most difficult question exercise
  4.15 Closing exercise
  4.30 Close

Day Four
  9.30 Opening exercise
  9.45 Practice presentation
 11.00 Coffee
 11.15 Practice presentation
 12.30 Lunch
  1.30 Practice presentation
  2.45 Tea
  3.00 Review of course and future planning
  4.15 Closing exercise

If outside speakers are to be invited to contribute to the programme, it is important to meet them during the pre-course planning stage. This provides a chance to agree what is required, to clarify the aims of their input and to discuss how it fits in with the rest of the course. The sort of outside speaker who may be particularly helpful on a course such as this would be a prison officer who is involved in HIV education and able to discuss the experience at another prison. On a practical level it is important to remember to let the prison gate staff know who is expected, and when, in advance so that time is not wasted on the day of the course.

The trainers may find it useful to draw up a more detailed course timetable for their own use. The purpose of this is to describe who is running each session, timings, methods to use, what resources will be necessary, and details of issues and outcomes expected from each exercise.

Example of Trainer's Timetable of the Course

Day One

Time	Lead	Method	Materials	Issues and Outcomes
9.30	RT	Welcome and introduction to the course		Participants will have a clearer idea of what they can expect from the course
9.35	JP	Name game: each participant says the name they wish to be known by etc.	Flip chart marker pens	Course leaders and participants become familiar with one another's names etc.

Negotiation with the Staff Training Department

Once agreement is reached with management about running staff training within the prison, more detailed negotiation needs to take place with the prison's training department. This should happen at the same time as the course planning process. The training department can arrange for the course to be advertised. It may help to provide them with a clear unambiguous poster describing the course, who it is aimed at, length, venue and where to get more information (see suggestion below). The training department will recruit and select the officers and it is useful to encourage them to include female and black staff if possible. In many male prisons female staff, and in all prisons black staff, are under-represented in the workforce and this is likely to be reflected in the make-up of the course membership.

**DO YOU WANT TO BECOME AN
HIV/AIDS TRAINER?**

A four-day training course for officers interested in taking on the education of colleagues and inmates about HIV and AIDS will be held from (date) to (date) at (location). If you would like to be involved in this important and challenging area of work please contact ....
in the Training Department. No previous knowledge or experience necessary. *Places are limited!*

Course trainers are employed by the Standing Conference on Drug Abuse.

Once participants have been selected, it is useful for them to be sent a letter of acceptance and a course programme. The trainers can do this themselves or they can ask the training officer if he or she will do it. A full list of names and staff locations (obtained from the training officer) will be needed to send details to all participants. It is important that course details are sent out in good time to allow staff on holiday/rest days to receive them. It may be helpful to restate the aims of the course in the letter to avoid misunderstanding. At some prisons staff may attend training in civilian clothes. The training officer should explain local practice. If it is possible for civilian clothes to be worn, this should be made explicit in the letter of acceptance.

Prisons usually have facilities that can be used for training. If these are to be used it is important to make arrangements with the training department to view them in advance of the course and to check out toilet, tea, coffee and lunch facilities, and to ensure that there will be no interruptions during the training. It is also useful to find out if the training department can supply any learning aids needed, e.g. flipchart and paper, video, overhead projector, pens.

Evaluation

A course should be evaluated against its original aims and objectives, the purpose being to assess whether the course has met its goals. There are two elements to this: evaluation of what happened during the course, and of what happens as a result of the course.

Any type of evaluation needs to include contributions from the trainers as well as the participants. The evaluation may be performed by the trainers, but there are obvious advantages in using an independent evaluator, or at least someone else from the outside agency involved, who may be perceived as being a little more independent. Taken together, information from both trainers and participants will provide feedback about how the course went, the effectiveness of individual exercises and the trainer's style. It can also provide information as to what changes, if any, would be advisable on future courses. It may be useful to write up these evaluations and keep a record that can be referred to. The prison may also request a summary.

The usual method of gaining feedback from participants is to hand out questionnaires at the end of the course, either asking that they be filled in before people leave or requesting that participants return them by post. A stamped addressed envelope may increase the number of returns if they are to be posted. The kind of questions that can be included in such a questionnaire fall into three categories:

(a) those which address the process of the course;
(b) those which relate to the aims and objectives;
(c) those which are knowledge based.

The questions asked may be fairly broad to enable the course participants to give their own impressions and the issues that arose for them.

Examples of the first type of question might be:

● What were the three main things you learned on the course?
● Were there any topics or issues that made you feel uncomfortable?
● What part of the course did you find least useful?
● How helpful were the trainers?
● How useful were the handouts provided?
● Is there anything that could be changed which would have made participating better for you?

Other questions might be directed at the adequacy of the practical arrangements, such as the location or times.

Questions aimed at trying to determine how well the course met its aims and objectives might take the following form:

● What skills, if any, do you feel you gained from participating in the course?
● How important is it to know the difference between HIV and AIDS? Why?
● What do you think are the three most important messages to include in an introductory session on HIV for staff?

As well as asking questions, a list of statements could be prepared, asking for the extent of agreement or disagreement with each.

For example:

● I feel confident enough to talk about sex.

- Talking about HIV and AIDS involves tackling people's prejudices.
- I find it easy to talk to other prison staff about HIV and AIDS.

A briefer approach might be simply to ask the participants how well the course met its objectives. This could be in the form of an open-ended question like: How well do you think the course met its objectives?

To evaluate changes in knowledge and attitudes resulting from the course it may be useful to arrange to conduct interviews with participants before and after the training. Where possible, it is advisable to use evaluators other than the trainers so that this process does not appear to be like a test which course participants either pass or fail but is clearly an element in evaluating the course.

Examples of questions to put to participants before and after the training might be:

- Do you think any of the inmates you have contact with might be HIV positive?
- What sort of symptoms would you expect to see?
- Some people have argued that all inmates should be tested for HIV on admission. Do you agree or disagree? Why?
- If an inmate is tested for HIV should officers in the wing or unit be told the result? Why?/Why not?
- Do you think inmates are at a high risk of contracting HIV?
- Do you think anyone you know socially is at risk of contracting HIV?

If a pre- and post-course evaluation is to be conducted it may be as well to arrange the first interview a couple of weeks before the course and the second a couple of weeks after it so that pre-existing attitudes and retention of the information beyond the immediate impact of the course are examined. The issue of anonymity of evaluation responses should be carefully considered. Although it may be desirable, it might be difficult to achieve in a prison setting when the numbers trained are small.

In general it is advisable to ensure that any evaluation questionnaire is brief and that it includes questions that will assist in the assessment of the current course as well as future course design. Further information about evaluating HIV education may be found in *Monitoring and Evaluating Local HIV/AIDS Health Promotion: a Review of Theory and Practice* (Moody *et al.*, 1991).

Maintaining the Momentum

At the end of a training course participants are often fired with enthusiasm. This can easily dissipate if the education package cannot be started immediately. To maintain interest and contact, trainers could adopt some of the following strategies:

- Encourage the prison to form a multi-disciplinary HIV/AIDS committee to co-ordinate educational initiatives;
- Encourage the trained officers to see themselves as a group and stay in contact with one another after the course;
- Encourage the group to nominate someone to act as a liaison officer or co-ordinator;
- Encourage the educator group to negotiate for practice days after the course to refine the package or to look at other information needed;
- Send a monthly letter to the group members providing an update on HIV and AIDS, community contacts and information about useful leaflets, posters, publications, training courses or conferences;
- Encourage contacts with staff in other prisons doing similar work;
- Send a questionnaire to participants three or six months after the course asking what has happened since, what problems they have encountered and what could help them;
- Check with management as to whether they thought the course was useful and ask them what plans they have for the training group.

Summary

Important elements in organising HIV training for staff in a prison include:

- setting clear aims and objectives for the training, and ensuring that they are shared with the prison, from the outset;
- ensuring that the trainers have a good knowledge of HIV and AIDS and the related issues of discrimination and risk reduction and are able to discuss sex, sexuality, drug use and race;
- assessing training needs and establishing the prevailing climate in the prison in relation to HIV and AIDS;
- extensive and detailed pre-course planning including discussion between the trainers of attitudes to different issues likely to be raised;

- negotiation with the prison's training department to ensure that the training course is advertised appropriately and that adequate training facilities can be made available;
- evaluation of the course by both trainers and participants;
- the development of a strategy to enable the officer/educators to receive support in their education work and up-to-date information.

Chapter 4

The Exercises

A Guide to the Exercises   39
Dealing with Difficult Issues   39

Name Game   41
Opening and Closing Exercises   42
Ground Rules   44
Expectations Exercise   46
Sorting the Facts from the Myths   48
Attitude Statement Exercise   50
Moral Dilemmas Role Play   52
Prison Situation Exercise   55
Drug Use Exercise   58
Safer Sex Exercise   61
Discussion on Training Methods   64
Devising an HIV Education Package   65
Difficult Question Carousel   68
Pair Work   71
Practising Presentations   72
Action Planning Exercise   74

A Guide to Using Handouts   76

A Guide to the Exercises

This chapter contains outlines of the exercises which comprise the Project's HIV awareness and training for educators course for prison officers. They are exercises that have worked in the prisons in which they have been used so far. Many are adapted from existing training packs (see Appendix 4), some are original. They are offered as suggestions which can be altered to suit a specific situation or used as a basis for creating other exercises.

When designing a course it is useful to build into the programme a wide range of activities so that participants are not sitting passively for long periods. The exercises described demand a high level of participation with an emphasis on confirming existing knowledge and learning from one another. The opportunity to work in small groups and pairs develops group members' relationships with one another and seems to facilitate group identity. We have found it useful for the trainers to ensure that individual participants do not work with the same small group throughout the course. Approximate timings have been given.

The following processes have been included in every course we have designed and we regard them as essential elements:

● Introductions to enable participants to get to know one another;
● Discussion and agreement on the principles on which the group will operate. This is usually achieved through a ground rule exercise;
● Time to explore ways of putting what has been learned on the course into practice. This is often done by means of an action planning exercise.

Instructions for running the exercises are based on the assumption that two trainers will be working together, and that they will have a good knowledge of HIV and AIDS and related issues. *Basic information about HIV is not included in the instructions for the exercises.*

Dealing with Difficult Issues

The 'Sorting the Facts from the Myths', 'Attitude Statement' and 'Prison Situation' exercises all include examples of statements and situations which the Project has used successfully. They are not intended as an exhaustive list and trainers may wish to design their own in order to raise specific issues. The statements in both the 'Sorting the Facts from the Myths' and 'Attitude Statement' exercises reflect the misinformation and prejudice which are often prevalent. Both the statements and scenarios are intended to provoke discussion and enable the course participants to explore the issues and marshal their own arguments to respond when they are in the role of educators. The issues they raise are complex, highly sensitive and controversial. It is important that the trainers spend time in advance of the course considering how best to handle them. One way to achieve this may be for the trainers to work through each statement or situation to be used, discussing issues that could come up. If necessary a more experienced HIV trainer could be asked to help by identifying with the course trainers areas likely to be raised. If discussion or disagreement occurs between the trainers it should be resolved *before the course starts*. Reference to the many books available about HIV and AIDS may help. Two which may prove particularly helpful are: *AIDS: Scientific and Social Issues* (Aggleton *et al.*, 1989), which contains factual information and explores prevailing beliefs about HIV and AIDS; *AIDS, Africa and Racism* by Richard and Rosalind Chirimuuta (1989), which challenges the powerful myth that AIDS originated in Africa. In addition, trainers may find it helpful to contact any of the national HIV and AIDS organisations listed in Appendix 6, to clarify any points which are causing confusion.

Attempting to change attitudes and correct misinformation about HIV and AIDS can be a daunting task since there are many grey areas. Careful attention to the preparation of the training course in general and these issues in particular will help it to run smoothly. Even with the best of ground work it is impossible to predict all the issues and questions which may arise from the prepared statements and situations. Course trainers should not be afraid to admit when they don't know the answer to a question or point raised during the course. In response it may be helpful to find out any relevant information and come back to the point later in the course if time permits or contact the course member who wanted the information after the course. Alternatively, course members can be referred to other sources of information (an integral part of the course – see Action Planning exercise) and many of these are listed in the appendices.

Name Game

Aims and Objectives
- To introduce participants and trainers to each other by name and to act as an icebreaker.

Materials
Flip chart, paper, marker pens.

Time
15–20 minutes.

Method
The group sits in a circle with a flip chart and pens placed in the centre. Each member of the group writes their name on the paper and says a couple of things about their name, e.g. whether they like it, why they were given it. To get this process going it is best if one of the facilitators starts. It may be helpful to stick the sheet of paper with all the names on the wall for the rest of the day.

Issues and Outcomes
- This can be a relaxed and friendly way to start off the process of getting to know one another and remembering each other's names.

Opening and Closing Exercises

Aims and Objectives
● To give everyone an opportunity to say something at the beginning and at the end of each day.
● To help participants to focus their minds on the day ahead and get to know each other again as a group.
● To give participants an opportunity to reflect on how the day has gone.

Time
About five minutes.

Method
The group is seated in a large circle for both exercises. One trainer gives the group a sentence to complete. The other trainer finishes the sentence first followed by the person either on her/his right or left until everyone has had a turn, finishing with the trainer who started the sentence. The group then moves on to the next part of the programme if it is an opening exercise or disperses after a closing exercise.

Here are some examples of the sort of incomplete sentence which could be used:

Opening
One thing I like about my job is . . .
One thing I dislike about my job is . . .
If I wasn't a prison officer, I would like to be . . .
The thing I am looking forward to on the course today is . . .

Closing
I enjoyed today because . . .
One thing I learned today was . . .
When I get home I'm going to . . .

Hints

Another way of running these exercises is to encourage participants to speak when they feel ready instead of going round the group from person to person.

It may be helpful to prepare sentences in advance; alternatively, they can be invented on the day so as to be more topical or relevant to specific issues and to the group.

If a participant chooses to raise an important issue during a brief opening or closing exercise trainers may wish either to acknowledge it and make space for it or ensure that it is addressed properly at another point on the course.

Issues and Outcomes

- These exercises can help to start and end the day on a positive note.
- Participants can decide whether to say something humorous or serious, to disclose something personal or be vague.
- This can be a useful way of receiving feedback as to how the course is being experienced by the participants.

Ground Rules

Aims and Objectives
- To encourage group members to agree on a set of principles which will help them to work together, be physically comfortable and feel relaxed.
- To create a supportive working environment in which participants can gain maximum benefit from the course.

Materials
Flip chart, paper, marker pens, note paper and pens for participants.

Time
Method 1: 15 minutes. Method 2: 20–45 minutes.

Method 1
A list of ground rules is presented on the flip chart by the trainer.

The trainer leads a discussion and encourages the group to agree on any additions or deletions to the list. It is displayed in a prominent position for the duration of the course so that it can be referred to if necessary.

Method 2
The trainer asks the participants to think individually about how they want to work together.

The group is encouraged to think individually of a group situation they have been in and to consider what stopped them from contributing, made them feel uncomfortable or created a good atmosphere. Participants are asked to write these down. If there are any difficulties the trainer may give an example. *(5 minutes)*

Participants form small groups of three or four and produce a list of rules they think are important. The notes they make individually can be used to help start discussion in the group. *(10 minutes)*

The small groups return to the large group and feed back the lists they have produced. The trainer then leads a discussion on these and encourages the group to reach a consensus. *(10 minutes)*

The list is displayed as in method 1.

> **Example of a list of ground rules**
> - All members to respect time keeping, i.e. start at 9.30, finish at 16.30 and return promptly from breaks.
> - Everyone to have a chance to speak *if they want to.*
> - Respect other people's contributions.
> - No smoking during sessions.
> - Wash up own cups.
> - Contributions to be confidential to the group in which they are made.

Issues and Outcomes

- This exercise should help participants to develop a self-structured framework within which work can take place.
- Group members are likely to be reassured if they have first had an opportunity to discuss and agree the way the group is to operate.
- Trainers need to discuss beforehand how they will handle situations where the rules are broken. For example: two people are missing at the start of an afternoon session. The trainers may remind the group about the punctuality rule and decide with the group either to start without them or wait a few minutes. The latecomers should be welcomed and made aware of their lateness but not humiliated.
- Confidentiality can have many meanings. Trainers need to be sure it is included in the list of rules and clearly defined so that participants understand what it means to them on the course. One way to define it is to say that personal disclosures or contributions are confidential to the group (whole group, small group or pair) and also to the moment in which they are made (so if someone is absent from a session he or she should not be told details later). The group may need to spend a few minutes exploring the sort of things which should be kept confidential.
- Confidentiality is an important issue in prisons. It is relevant to give particular focus to it in this exercise because:
– it will probably come up several times during the course;
– participants who come from the same prison need to be assured that their contributions will not be talked about outside the group;
– the course aims to address sensitive issues such as sex, drug use and the manner in which prisoners with HIV are dealt with.
- Ground rules may help to prevent conflict occurring within the group.
- They can be modified if necessary to help the course to run smoothly.

Expectations Exercise

Aims and Objectives
- To clarify what participants expect to gain from the course.
- To highlight any specific issues that people might want to raise during the course.

Materials
Flip chart, marker pens, note paper and pens for participants.

Time
30 minutes.

Method
The group divides into pairs to identify the main things they hope to gain from the course. *(5 minutes)*

The pairs then form into small groups of four and, as a group, develop a list of their common personal and professional expectations of the course. *(10 minutes)*

The large group re-forms and each small group feeds back their main expectations.

These can be put on a flip chart by the trainer and prioritised by the group. *(15 minutes)*

Hint
The time required to run this exercise can be reduced by excluding the small group stage.

Issues and Outcomes
- This exercise allows participants to clarify what they want out of the course. It gives an opportunity for people to raise specific issues which they want highlighted. It also allows for unrealistic expectations to be identified.

● A range of expectations may come up, some of which may not be covered in the course. It is useful if trainers know where people can find out more information.

● It may be necessary to make it clear that this is not an agenda setting exercise. Obviously, particular issues can be given greater emphasis if participants so wish, but if the course programme has already been set it may be difficult to include entirely new issues.

Sorting the Facts from the Myths

Aims and Objectives
● To present basic information about HIV and AIDS, the routes of transmission, the difference between HIV and AIDS, and methods of preventing HIV infection.
● To dispel myths and to begin to correct misinformation about HIV and AIDS.

Materials
Prepared cards, each with a typed statement about HIV or AIDS. About 30 will be needed for a group of 12 people.

Flip chart, paper, marker pens, Blu-tack.

Here are some examples of the sort of statements which could be used:

Babies can catch AIDS from their mothers.

HIV can be passed on by sweat, urine and tears.

You can become infected with HIV if someone who has the virus bites you.

Having a negative test result means that HIV is not present.

There is no risk of becoming infected with HIV by giving artificial respiration.

HIV originated in Africa.

Sharing injecting equipment can spread HIV.

Heterosexual sex cannot pass on HIV.

Oral sex is a form of safer sex.

Many opportunistic infections can be successfully treated.

Note: Please refer to 'Dealing with Difficult Issues' at the beginning of this chapter before using this exercise.

Time
About 90 minutes.

Method

Participants divide into groups of three or four. Six or seven cards are distributed to each group plus a sheet of flip chart paper divided into three columns: 'True', 'False' and 'Don't Know'. Each group is asked to reach a consensus on the best column in which to place each card and then attach them with Blu-tack to the appropriate column. *(30 minutes)*

The large group reassembles and discusses why each card in turn is so placed. *(60 minutes)*

Hints

Statements on the cards in this exercise may usefully concentrate on 'facts' (be they true or false) rather than attitudes if the attitude exercises are to appear later in the course. Participants often seem to value some solid knowledge at an early stage.

Cards in the 'Don't Know' column usually produce the most discussion. *It may help to discuss these first.*

Each group should talk about a card they have discussed, then the next group and so on. This helps to maintain interest.

It may be useful to include a short talk before doing this exercise which focuses on the routes of transmission, difference between HIV and AIDS, and methods of prevention of HIV infection. This can be followed by a question-and-answer session. It allows participants to start this exercise with a little more confidence.

Issues and Outcomes

● The group will have an opportunity to distinguish facts from prejudice and misinformation.

● This exercise provides an opportunity for participants to test out their knowledge and develop their arguments in small groups before arguing the point with the larger group.

● Trainers have the chance to highlight several key points which are likely to arise repeatedly during the discussion, e.g. you can't catch AIDS; HIV and AIDS are not interchangeable terms.

Attitude Statement Exercise

Aims and Objectives
● To identify the various influences that can affect attitudes and values concerning HIV and AIDS.
● To begin to examine some of the social, economic and political aspects of HIV and AIDS.

Materials
Prepared cards, each with a statement about HIV or AIDS written on it. About 25 cards should be prepared though they will not all be needed. One bin, box or plastic bag to put the cards in.

Examples of useful statements follow. The discussion can be made very topical through the design of further statements.

Africans and Haitians are high-risk groups.

Safer sex should be taught in schools.

If you have HIV it is better to know about it.

AIDS is God's punishment for people who are deviant.

Women should take prime responsibility for safer sex.

Injecting drug users cannot avoid HIV infection.

Everyone should be tested for HIV and those who have it should be sent to a special place where they could be isolated and live out their lives in comfort.

Not enough resources are available to educate people about HIV and AIDS.

Haemophiliacs and children are the innocent victims of the AIDS epidemic.

It is advisable for a woman who is HIV antibody positive to have an abortion.

Note: Please refer to 'Dealing with Difficult Issues' at the beginning of this chapter before using this exercise.

Time
60 minutes.

Method

The container with cards inside is placed on the floor in the middle of the group.

Each person takes a card in turn, reads it out and shares their initial reaction with the group. The group then discusses issues raised by the statement before the next participant takes a card.

Hints

Another way of running this exercise is for participants to take a card when they want to, rather than going round each in turn. It may be helpful for one of the trainers to go first to give the group an idea what is expected.

It is unlikely that everyone will get a turn. This exercise can be returned to if there is any spare time later in the course.

Time on each statement may be limited but it is important that there is sufficient space for more considered discussion to follow the initial reaction.

Issues and Outcomes

• Participants will have the opportunity to consider a range of opinions, some of which may challenge their own view.

• It is not possible to discuss issues such as homophobia, sexism, racism and drug use in depth in one hour. Some issues may crop up again at other points during the course where they can be explored more fully. Information around the issues raised can be made available to course participants wishing to pursue them further. Trainers should consider in advance how they wish to deal with this.

• The exercise should allow group members to be clear that it is high-risk behaviour which can lead to the transmission of HIV and that the idea of high-risk groups is spurious.

• HIV and AIDS affect everyone. This exercise demonstrates that it is not just a medical issue but affects every sphere of life.

Moral Dilemmas Role Play

Aims and Objectives
- To explore some of the attitudes demonstrated towards people affected by HIV and AIDS. The non-prison setting is designed to enable this to happen in an objective manner away from the pressures which are sometimes engendered by HIV in prison.
- To experience the demands and tensions of making decisions in a different role.

Materials
Three different versions of a situation typed on separate sheets.

1. You are the school governors of a primary school in Greentop, a village on the outskirts of a large town. The school is the only one in the village and public transport links with the nearest town are poor, so all the village children attend your school. A new family have recently moved from the town into the village and they want to send their six-year-old son Peter Adams to the school. There are rumours around that both parents are ex-drug users and that Peter is HIV positive. The local paper has just been in touch to ask if Peter is to be allowed to attend the school. They said they had heard he 'has AIDS' from contacts in the area the family moved from. You are holding a meeting to discuss the situation.

2. You are all parents of children attending the primary school in Greentop, a village on the outskirts of a large town. Since there is no good bus service to the town and the school is the only one in the village, all the village children attend the same school. A new family have recently moved from the town to the village. They have a six-year-old son Peter Adams who, you have heard, is going to start at the school. The local paper had a reporter outside the school gates yesterday afternoon talking to people waiting to collect their children. He said that Peter's parents are 'junkies' and that Peter 'has AIDS'. You are having a meeting in the village hall to discuss the situation.

3. You are a team of social workers for an area which includes the village of Greentop. It is a close-knit community which can be hostile to

newcomers. You have recently had a referral from your colleagues in the nearest town. The family concerned have just moved to Greentop. John Adams, the father of the family, is an ex-drug user, though Elspeth, his wife, is not. However, he contracted HIV in the early 1980s and unwittingly passed it on to Elspeth. Neither was aware they had the infection until after the birth of their son Peter six years ago. Fortunately, tests have shown that Peter did not acquire HIV from Elspeth before his birth. The family faced considerable local hostility at their last address and that is why they moved. The local paper there had been responsible for stirring up prejudice. The social services are involved because of the family's need for support and because Peter is becoming very withdrawn and shy since no other children have been allowed to play with him. Your task is to help the family, and Peter in particular, to settle into the village and the school. You are having a team meeting to decide how you can do this without breaking confidentiality. All seemed to be going well until you heard that the local paper had started to take an interest in the family.

Time
About 90 minutes.

Method
Participants are divided into three groups. One group will be school governors, one parents and the third social workers, though they should not be told this in advance. The appropriate story sheets are distributed to the groups and each person is asked to read their version at least twice. Each group discusses their situation and develops a plan of action. *(20 minutes)*

The large group then re-forms for feedback which can be led in various ways. It is useful to ask each group to present their feedback and then encourage a general discussion between the groups while still in role. This can then be followed by a general discussion out of role on how the exercise felt and the issues it raised. *(70 minutes)*

Hints
It may help the 'social workers' to feed back last as this is a particularly difficult role to play.

[continued

No participant has the whole story during the exercise. This is deliberate in the design of the exercise and true to situations in real life. If participants feel it is artificial, it may be helpful to acknowledge it and encourage them to stay in role.

Issues and Outcomes

● Some themes which may emerge:
– the way attitudes can be shaped by stereotypes;
– parents should know the facts about HIV, AIDS and drugs and educate their children;
– the local health authority should educate the school governors and staff;
– the main responsibility of the social workers is to support the family;
– parents' worries about their children 'catching AIDS' at the school;
– the meaning of confidentiality and what to do when it is breached.

● The people at the centre of this situation, Peter, John and Elspeth, are not given a voice in this exercise. It may be worth considering their inclusion as a fourth group if numbers allow, though they would require a 'story sheet' to be written for them. However, the fact that they are not there to be asked for 'facts' can be quite powerful. People with HIV are often deprived of a voice when prejudices are being aired and decisions made about them.

Prison Situation Exercise

Aims and Objectives

● To apply knowledge about HIV and AIDS to everyday situations faced by staff and prisoners in and out of prison.

● To identify personal reactions and attitudes to situations and how they might affect professional practice.

Materials

Prepared cards with brief outlines of a situation written on each. About 12 cards should be prepared for a group of 12 people.

Examples

You notice that a prisoner on your landing has been losing weight rapidly, suffers from night sweats and complains of pain in his neck, armpits and groin. When you suggest he sees the prison doctor he just says he is feeling a bit under the weather and that it will pass.
    What is your reaction? What do you do?

You are a male prison officer. A new female officer has just arrived at the prison. One night you are both at a disco at the officers' club and you give her a lift home. She asks you in and it becomes obvious that she is as interested in you as you are in her. As you are about to get into bed you get your condoms out of your pocket but she says 'It's OK, I'm on the pill.'
    What is your reaction? What do you do?

You are in the kitchen. A cook cuts himself badly while chopping some meat. He bleeds profusely. To stop the bleeding an officer wraps a tea towel around the wound. A prisoner begins to clear up the blood with a dish cloth.
    What is your reaction? What do you do?

You are on duty one evening and a colleague, who is also a close friend, approaches you and asks if he can talk to you about something personal. He tells you that he has recently been to a GUM clinic and was tested for HIV. The result was positive. He wants to know whether you think he should tell his wife.
    What is your reaction? What do you do?

You are on duty as landing officer and a prisoner you have known for several months approaches you and asks for some advice. His pregnant girlfriend told him during a visit two weeks ago that she has HIV. She says that she has always been faithful to him, even while he has been in prison.
    What is your reaction? What do you do?

While you are watching TV one evening your partner enters the room looking a bit anxious and holding some papers from a training course you are attending about HIV and AIDS. He or she says, 'I don't see why you have to know about HIV and AIDS. Surely only the hospital officers should have to deal with people with HIV or AIDS?'
    What is your reaction? What do you do?

[Continued

You regularly work on a remand landing with several injecting drug users on it. Although frequent searches are conducted and nothing has been found, you are fairly sure they have access to a needle and syringe which they probably share. A new prisoner has just arrived accompanied by a police form saying he was withdrawing from heroin while in their custody and has HIV. He is an assertive individual who knows how to cope in prison. It is likely he will make contact with the other drug users quickly.

What is your reaction? What do you do?

You approach a long-term prisoner, well known for his violence and sexual activity in prison, to ask if he wants to come to your HIV education session. He says, 'I don't believe in HIV or AIDS. It's all a media conspiracy.' You know that he regularly forces younger men to have unsafe sex with him though nobody complains for obvious reasons.

What is your reaction? What do you do?

During slop-out you overhear two prisoners talking in the recess about another prisoner who is about to be transferred back from the hospital. The rumour is that this person has been seriously ill due to AIDS. They are discussing whether or not to organise a protest to stop him coming to the wing.

What is your reaction? What do you do?

You are discussing how you got on at an HIV and AIDS training course held in the prison last week over lunch in the mess. A principal officer sitting nearby says in your hearing '. . . well, we all know it's gay men and drug users who are responsible for spreading AIDS. I don't see why we need a course about it in here.'

What is your reaction? What do you do?'

You are requested to do a cell search with a colleague. During the search your colleague is gently moving some clothes off a bed when something pricks his finger which makes it bleed. You carefully sort through the clothes and discover a needle and syringe.

What is your reaction? What do you do?

You are a prisoner who has just been transferred from another prison. You know you are HIV positive but you did not dare tell anyone at the last prison as you wanted to be on normal location. Others told you that once you say you are HIV positive, the whole prison finds out, making life very difficult. During reception at the new prison you are shown a paper which says that confidentiality is maintained and that people who are HIV positive and well are kept on normal location. Discreet medical checks to monitor health are available via the daily sick parade.

What is your reaction? What do you do?

Note: Please refer to 'Dealing with Difficult Issues' at the beginning of this chapter before using this exercise.

Time
90 minutes.

Method
Participants are divided into groups of three or four. Three cards are distributed to each group.

The groups read the cards and discuss their initial reactions and then what they would do about each situation. *(30 minutes)*

Each group then gives a brief résumé of their discussion in the large group followed by general discussion on the issues raised. *(60 minutes)*

Hint
If the groups each feed back one situation in turn it helps the discussion to flow and maintains interest.

Issues and Outcomes
● This exercise can highlight the differences between personal attitudes and responses to situations and the expectations of professional roles within prison.

● It reinforces some of the information contained in the facts exercises and the video *AIDS Inside and Out.*

● Some issues raised in this exercise:
– the treatment of prisoners living with HIV and AIDS;
– the need for prisons to have an HIV and AIDS policy;
– prisoners' access to specialist counselling;
– the need to educate staff and prisoners about HIV and AIDS;
– the different attitudes of staff towards prisoners in general and drug users in particular;
– the conflict prison staff may experience between their role of maintaining security and addressing the welfare needs of prisoners;
– attitudes, to and possibly conflict with, current government policy of not supplying condoms or clean injecting equipment to prisoners.

Drug Use Exercise

Aims and Objectives
● To increase awareness of legal and illegal drugs.
● To highlight the ways in which drug use may be connected to HIV transmission.
● To introduce the concept of risk reduction.

Materials
Flip chart paper divided into two columns, marker pens. Syringes and needles – sufficient for one per three people. These can be obtained from chemists and drug agencies. Plastic or paper cups, water, bleach (not chlorine-free bleach which is ineffective for this purpose), washing up liquid. Sharps box for safe disposal of syringes and needles (available from drug agencies).

Time
About 75 minutes.

Method
Participants divide into pairs. Each pair writes the names of as many drugs as they can think of in the left-hand column. (5 minutes)

Pairs then discuss whether use of each drug listed is likely to carry any risk of HIV transmission and write this in the right-hand column. (High, medium, low or none.) *(10 minutes)*

The large group reconvenes and discusses the issues raised. *(45 minutes)*

During the discussion it may be useful to ensure that drugs in prison and the treatment of drug users in prison are mentioned. After exploring the difficulties and reflecting on the notion of risk reduction, participants are likely to be ready for the next stage.

The trainers then demonstrate how to clean a syringe and needle and dispose of them safely.

Each person then has an opportunity to clean a syringe and needle correctly. *(15 minutes)*

Detailed instructions on how to clean needles and syringes are not included here. These can be obtained from drug agencies and syringe and needle exchange schemes. County lists of these are available from SCODA. They may also help you with any training you need before demonstrating to others.

Hint

When participants are listing drugs it may be helpful to suggest that they describe types of drug (e.g. tranquillisers) rather than a multitude of brand names. Otherwise this exercise can become rather competitive.

Prison officers are well aware that security strategies such as searching have limited impact on the use of drugs in prison. The idea of cleaning needles and syringes may be best presented after some careful ground work on risk reduction during the discussion because the whole idea is likely to be unfamiliar to participants.

If needles and syringes are taken into a prison for this exercise it is important that they are all accounted for and removed after the session.

Issues and Outcomes

● Trainers need to be clear about the aims and objectives of including the practical syringe and needle cleaning part of this exercise. Some questions worth considering with the group are:

– Injecting drug use does happen in prison but is illegal. Is it ethical to give information to prisoners on how to clean a prohibited item? Is it ethical not to when this may reduce their risk of contracting HIV?

– Is it valid, given that prisoners do not have easy access at present to substances such as bleach which are known to deactivate HIV? Washing up liquid and other detergents do not deactivate the virus but help to rid the syringe and needle of blood which may contain the virus.

● It is important to ensure that both legal and illegal drugs are covered in the discussion. In particular it is useful to focus on alcohol as a significant factor in the transmission of HIV because of its disinhibiting effects.

● Other issues that can be discussed in this exercise are:

– different ways drugs can be taken;

– different uses to which drugs can be put. It is important to include

[continued

drugs in sport and recreational use;
– different types of people who might take drugs;
– risk reduction strategies relating to HIV.

Safer Sex Exercise

Aims and Objectives
- To introduce the basic idea of safer sex activities.
- To discuss how a safer sex message can be appropriately communicated in a prison setting.

Materials
Condoms, latex squares (known as dental dams or oral shields), flip chart paper, biros and marker pens, index cards, plastic bag or other container for cards, Blu-tack.

Time
About 75 minutes.

Method
Participants are asked, working alone, to complete this statement on an index card: 'My dictionary definition of safer sex is . . .' *(3 minutes)*

The large group reconvenes and all the cards are placed in the container. Each person picks out a card. If this card is the definition he/she wrote, it is put back into the container and an alternative one is selected. Each person reads out the card they have picked and shares their reaction. Other people may comment but it is best not to have a group discussion at this stage. *(25 minutes)*

Participants divide into groups of three or four. The groups list as many sexual activities as they can. Each group selects five of these and writes each on a card. *(5 minutes)*

The small groups then discuss how to order these in a hierarchy from 'No/lowest risk' to 'Highest risk'. They are attached with Blu-tack on to a continuum line drawn on flip chart paper.

An example of the result might be

No/lowest Risk	MASSAGE	MUTUAL MASTURBATION	ORAL SEX WITH A CONDOM OR DENTAL DAM	VAGINAL SEX WITH A CONDOM	UNPROTECTED ANAL SEX	*Highest Risk*

(10 minutes)

[continued

The flip chart sheets are placed on the floor or attached to a wall so that people can see what other groups have produced. The large group then discusses the issues raised in the small groups. *(30 minutes)*

Hints

It may be appropriate to start this exercise with a short introductory talk to give people some idea of what safer sex is. There is some useful information about safer sex contained in the book *Safer Sex: the Guide for Women Today* by D. Richardson. (See Bibliography.)

If possible, split the group into same sex small groups. This can be useful as many issues around safer sex are gender specific.

The condoms and latex squares can be handed round during the discussion and information given on how to use them.

Issues and Outcomes

● People may find this exercise difficult and produce lists which are very general. Encourage them to think about activities such as kissing rather than strategies such as monogamy.

● Human sexuality and safer sex is an enormous subject. Only basic ideas can be covered in this exercise. Some important areas worth considering are:

– sex can be difficult to talk about;

– people's understanding of what sex is can be different;

– the importance of not assuming that everyone is heterosexual or that everyone with HIV is gay or a drug user;

– safer sex can also be a way of reducing the risk of contracting other sexually transmitted diseases or becoming pregnant.

● Power imbalances in sexual situations need to be recognised by anyone passing on safer sex information. It may be difficult for prison officer/ educators to address this issue in great depth in a brief education session for prisoners, but it is important that the safer sex message acknowledges the problem of negotiating safer sex in such a situation and goes further than simply saying 'use a condom'.

● Prison staff should know how to protect themselves from the sexual transmission of HIV. Participants may discuss whether they believe that condoms and latex squares should/should not be made available to prisoners during their sentence and/or on release. They may also begin to think of creative and appropriate ways of putting across other aspects of safer sex to prisoners.

• It may be helpful for trainers to think about how they could handle any homophobic attitudes or comments made by participants *before* the course starts.

Discussion on Training Methods

Aims and Objectives
- To identify the training methods used on the course so far.
- To examine their usefulness in presenting information to prisoners and staff.

Materials
Handout on training methods (an example of a useful handout is provided in Appendix 2), flip chart and marker pen.

Time
30–45 minutes.

Method
The large group is asked to name or describe training methods used on the course so far. One trainer writes these on the flip chart. The handout is then distributed and any omissions rectified. The group is encouraged to identify which methods have been most effective and what other factors they will need to consider in designing training (for example, the aims of the training, type of group, likely size of group and time available).

Issues and Outcomes
- Participants will have the opportunity to identify the training methods used and to discuss those which have been most useful. This provides a starting point for designing an education package to be delivered by the course participants.
- This exercise marks the turning point where course members can start to see themselves as potential educators.

Devising an HIV Education Package

Aims and Objectives
- To identify the aims and objectives of an HIV education package.
- To devise an outline for a two-hour HIV education package for prisoners.
- To discuss how this package can be adapted for different groups such as prison staff.

Materials
Flip chart and marker pens.

Time
60–90 minutes.

Method
Participants divide into groups of four. Each group lists the KEY MESSAGES they want to communicate in the package.

They return to the large group to clarify the aims of the package. The trainer writes these on one sheet of the flip chart. *(15 minutes)*

They then return to the same groups.

Each group makes two lists of WHAT should be included in the package and HOW.

The large group re-forms and discusses the lists which are collated by the trainer as before. *(25 minutes)*

The large group devises one package from the versions produced in the small groups. One trainer leads the discussion. The other records the consensus reached on the flip chart which is then displayed. *(20–50 minutes)*

[continued

Example of a two-hour education package for prisoners produced by a group of prison officers

Introduction

Brainstorm in pairs on the difference between HIV and AIDS

Quiz on myths/facts about HIV/AIDS

Short introduction to *AIDS Inside and Out* video

Screening of video

Question-and-answer session

Go back to review answers in quiz

Break

Situation exercise in small groups about safer sex and drug use

Demonstration on how to clean a needle and syringe

Short presentation on where to get further information or counselling

Hints

Factors and questions often considered in developing a package include:
– people's concentration span: 20 minutes maximum?
– size of group: 8–16 maximum?
– how long for each part?
– is there a variety of activities to maintain interest?
– advertising of session: how, when, where?
– compulsory or voluntary attendance?
– length of session – one-and-a-half hours or two hours?
– timing: at induction, during sentence or as part of a pre-release course?
– will trainers be working in pairs?

It may be worth asking the group to identify the answers to these points by displaying a list of these questions on flip chart paper during the exercise.

Presenting accurate factual information about HIV in a brief and accessible form is a difficult task for anyone designing an HIV education package. One way around this is to suggest the use of the video *AIDS*

Inside and Out to provide the main factual input so that the officers can deal with discussion arising from it and other aspects, such as attitudes and risk reduction, in the rest of the package. In any event, it is useful to show this video at some point during the training of the officer/ educators. Every prison has a copy, but it is important to ask for it to be made available in advance since in prisons where it is not shown regularly it may need to be obtained from another department.

Issues and Outcomes

- It is helpful to break up this exercise into sections for small and large groups. This allows people to be creative and assists in developing a package which the group feels happy with.
- Participants should have identified how the exercises may be adapted to meet the differing needs of various groups of people. Not only will the education needs of staff differ from those of prisoners, but prisoners' needs will vary depending on the stage they have reached in their sentences. Similarly, women prisoners, young offenders and male prisoners will all require a different emphasis.

Note

A valuable addition to this exercise is to invite an officer who has experience in presenting an HIV education package in another prison to speak to the group. It can be encouraging for participants to hear that obstacles can be overcome and that prison officers can learn how to present a package with confidence and make improvements to it as they gain experience.

The reason why this exercise is about designing a two-hour package is that the available time for work, education, etc. in a prison morning or afternoon tends to be about two hours.

Difficult Question Carousel

Aims and Objectives
- To practice answering difficult questions on HIV and AIDS.
- To listen to the different ways in which these questions are answered.

Materials
One chair for each person.

Time
60 minutes.

Method
Each participant is asked to prepare a question, to be written down or memorised, about HIV and AIDS in prison. It can be a question likely to be asked by a prisoner or by a member of staff. It should be difficult, but not an impossible question to answer.

Half the participants place their chairs in a circle facing outwards. The second half place their chairs in a circle outside the first circle, each facing a member of the inner circle. This should result in two large circles so that people can easily talk to the person opposite without the distraction of others. Name the inner circle A and the outer circle B.

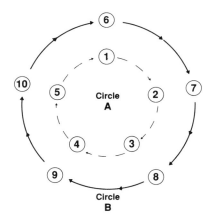

Each person in inner circle A asks the person opposite in circle B their question. Those in outer circle B give their answer. Allow about one-and-a-half minutes per question and answer. Then call 'change'.

People in circle B move round one chair in a clockwise direction. People in circle A ask the same question of the new person sitting opposite.

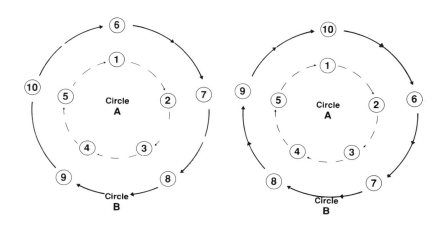

This sequence is repeated until circle A has asked everyone in circle B a question.

The process is then reversed. Circle B asks everyone in circle A their questions. Either circle A moves round this time or circle B as before.

A follow-up discussion is then led by a trainer in the large group. For example, the group can be asked what it felt like, what they noticed and whether they were surprised. It is not necessary to identify who asked or answered a specific question.

Suggestions for questions which might be asked if participants lack ideas:

Prisoner: 'Why can't I get bleach on the wing, guv?'

Prison officer: 'Why is there so much fuss about HIV and AIDS … what about all the mentally ill people banged up in here?'

Either: 'What would you do if I told you I'm HIV positive?'

[continued

Hints

This is usually a noisy exercise but can be fun. The time allowed can be shortened or lengthened as appropriate to achieve the aim of the exercise. The follow-up discussion should be brief. It may be useful to ask participants to start thinking of a difficult question earlier in the day on which this exercise is to take place.

Issues and Outcomes

● Participants have another opportunity to apply new knowledge or experience gained on the course so far by framing questions and answering them.

● They may experience difficulty in answering a question but learn positive ways of saying: 'I don't know but I'll try and find out and get back to you.'

● Some participants may choose to express to each other fears or doubts about HIV education within their prison.

● It can help people to anticipate some of the difficult questions they may be asked as educators when presenting the package to prisoners or during the course of their daily duties.

Pair Work

Aims and Objectives
- To prepare a presentation of one part of the education package designed during the course.
- To work in pairs applying theory to practice.

Materials
Have available: paper, flip chart, marker pens, training packs, information leaflets, cartoons, handouts distributed so far, books on HIV and AIDS.

Time
60 minutes or longer if possible.

Method
The group divides into pairs and selects which part they would like to present.

This is worked out so that everyone is happy and clear about their area of responsibility. The trainer writes names next to items on the programme and displays it for reference. Pairs begin their preparation.

Issues and Outcomes
- Some participants may express anxiety about giving a presentation if they have not done one before or because they are unsure how best to present new information. Trainers should be available for support, encouragement, and to point people to appropriate sources of information.
- Participants usually tackle this task with creativity and enthusiasm.
- This exercise follows on naturally from devising the HIV education package. If the presentations are to be given on the following day, it may be a good idea for people to have 15 minutes or so on that day to put final touches to their presentation or to ask the trainers questions.

Practising Presentations

Aims and Objectives

● To practise presenting one part of the education package designed during the course to the rest of the group.

● To receive feedback on the practice presentations.

Materials

Trainers should ensure that there is a good supply of: flip charts and paper, marker pens, cards, paper, biros.

If any equipment (such as an overhead projector, acetate sheets, video recorder, videos and television) is required it is a good idea to ensure that it is available and in good working order. It is advisable for participants to practise how to operate the equipment before the presentations so they feel confident.

Time

The following points need to be considered when planning the timings of the presentations. The aim is to ensure that each pair has sufficient time to present and receive feedback. Calculations should take account of:

– the number of participants;
– the number of components in the devised education package;
– the fact that some parts may need more time than others;
– the amount of time programmed.

Trainers may choose to explain how much time each group has and how timekeeping will be maintained.

Method

This is a suggested framework to facilitate positive feedback to the presenters. The aim is to give positive criticism and encouragement rather than negative or destructive comments.

1. At the end the presenters say how they felt about their presentations – whether they felt they communicated effectively and achieved their aims and objectives.

2. Other participants can then say what they learnt. Positive criticisms can be made *if requested by the presenters.*

3. Trainers make any specific comments on content and style. People who want more personal feedback should approach the trainers at the end of the session or on another occasion if more appropriate.

Each pair presents and receives feedback following the order of the devised education package.

It may happen that one or two pairs present the same part of the package. The group will have to decide whether to have these one after the other or placed elsewhere in the sequence.

Issues and Outcomes

● Once the group has seen the presentations they may decide to make some changes to the package. This may require a separate session so that the package has the essential elements but is also balanced. Course timings should take account of this.

● The presentations provide an opportunity to see how much knowledge has been retained.

● Participants are able to receive feedback on their performance so that they can make any necessary adjustments. The feedback may also boost the confidence of anyone who is feeling rather nervous about presenting the education sessions.

Action Planning Exercise

Aims and Objectives
● To review what has been gained on the course.
● To devise a personal and professional action plan.

Materials
Pens, paper, flip chart and paper, markers.

Time
About 60 minutes.

Method
Participants are asked to write down individually what they have gained from the course and what they would like to do next, personally and professionally, on HIV education. *(10 minutes)*

They then form pairs to discuss what they have written. *(5 minutes)*

The pairs join to form groups of four to formulate a list of professional goals. *(10 minutes)*

The large group then reconvenes and trainers take feedback from the groups. There may well be some consensus at this point and a useful way of organising the discussion (and notes on flip chart paper) may be by considering the following questions:
– What are they going to do?
– When are they going to do it?
– How are they going to do it?
– What/who may hinder?
– How can these hindrances be overcome?
– What/who may help?
– How can this help be obtained?
– Who is responsible for what?
– When should something be achieved by?

During the discussion the group may wish to draw up a joint action plan or spend five minutes working individually to formulate personal action plans. It may also be useful to set a time-scale for meeting again to review progress on these plans. *(35 minutes)*

Issues and Outcomes

• Further training needs may be identified. Information about courses, books, organisations and other resources can be made available.

• The group may feel that there should be someone within the prison to act as liaison officer between the group and the trainers for future contact.

• The group may express a need to practise the package further before presenting it to prisoners.

• The group may feel that a multi-disciplinary HIV/AIDS committee should be set up, if one is not already in existence, to encourage and develop the implementation of the education package within the prison.

• The participants may question the future role of the trainers at this stage. It would be advisable to work out beforehand the level of continuing support or contact, if any, to be offered. It may be most appropriate to leave the majority of the work to the officer/educators but to be involved in any review meeting planned and maintain low-level contact with any liaison officer or co-ordinator appointed.

A Guide to Using Handouts

For most of the course people actively participate in the learning process. Therefore there is not much opportunity, nor is it desirable, for participants to take notes. Because of this it can be useful to give handouts to the group to remind them of the main issues covered in an exercise. Course members often expect to be given something to read. It is our experience that many participants are highly motivated to learn and take the handouts home and read them overnight.

There are many types of handout: outlines of the main points covered in a short talk, magazine articles relevant to the topics covered, tables of facts and figures, diagrams of instructions, cartoons, and lists of further information and resources. When producing handouts it is worth considering the following points:

– They can take a long time to prepare and photocopy.
– Give thought to how and when they will be distributed to the group. For example, some handouts can be used during an exercise or referred to immediately afterwards. People generally start to read them once they are handed out, which will disturb their concentration. It may be useful to distribute handouts which are relevant to each day at the end of the day.
– Permission is usually required before photocopying from books, magazines and other printed material.

Here is an outline of some of the handouts produced by the Project for each day.

Day One
● outline of talk on basic facts about HIV and AIDS (given out after talks). Aggleton, P. *et al.* (1989) *AIDS: Scientific and Social Issues.* Churchill Livingstone, Edinburgh contains useful information for this, and for the illnesses and myths handouts;
● table of number of people with AIDS in the UK (published in *AIDS Dialogue*, see Appendix 7);
● description of AIDS-related illnesses;
● short descriptions dispelling myths about HIV and AIDS.

Day Two
- extracts from the Woolf Report on the management of HIV and AIDS and drug users in prisons (reproduced in Appendix 3);
- articles from newsletters and magazines about HIV, AIDS and prisons (there have been several articles in *AIDS Matters* and *Prison Service Journal* – see Appendix 7);
- statement on AIDS in prisons from the World Health Organisation (for copies write to: World Health Organisation, Global Programme on AIDS, Distribution and Sales, 20 Avenue Appia, 1211 Geneva, Switzerland. Title: 'Statement from the Consultation on Prevention and Control of AIDS in Prisons', ref: WHO/SPA/INF/87.14);
- poster of cartoon 'The A–Z of safer sex' (obtainable from the Lifeline Project Ltd, c/o North West Regional Drug Training Unit, Globe House, Southall Street, Manchester M3 1LG, price £1);
- instructions on how to clean a syringe and needle (contact Community Drug Project, 30 Manor Place, London SE17 3BB. Telephone 071-703 0559 for copies of their *User's Guide to Safer Drug Use*).

Day Three
- article from *Prison Service Journal* on the prison officer as an AIDS trainer (Clark, M. (1990) 'The prison officer as an AIDS trainer and counsellor', *Prison Service Journal*, No. 78, Spring);
- short description of training methods used on the course given out during the exercise (this handout was devised by Jan Mojsa and is reproduced in Appendix 2).

Day Four
- information on how to deliver presentations and deal with anxiety (refer to Mandel, S. (1988) *Effective Presentation Skills*, Kogan Page, London);
- list of information on organisations, magazines and books (see Appendices 4, 6 and 7 and the Bibliography).

Chapter 5

Other Initiatives in HIV and AIDS Education

Most people recognise that education and training are important in preventing the transmission of HIV both in prisons and in the wider community. Within British prisons there are now various initiatives which have been developed to provide basic information to staff and prisoners. There is considerable variety in the type, extent and influence of the work undertaken. While some prisons are still at the stage of identifying need, others have developed programmes that have moved on from providing basic information to considering the service needs of prisoners. The differences between establishments are on several levels:
– the extent to which the varied educational needs of prisoners and training needs of staff are being met;
– which department within the prison has been nominated as responsible for this work;
– the grade and number of staff involved;
– whether or not there is a multi-disciplinary HIV/AIDS committee;
– resource availability.

Despite every prison having been supplied with HIV educational packages, including videos, by the Prison Department, there are large differences in the extent to which there is any HIV education.

Another variable element is the level to which community-based health agencies, including the NHS, in either the drugs or HIV field have been involved in prison work. Community-based agencies have long been involved in working with prisoners. The main approaches are advice or counselling sessions, for individuals or groups, or involvement in prison-organised induction or pre-release sessions (NACRO, 1987).

Throughout the country many drug and HIV services are engaged in carrying out this type of work. They act as valuable supports to people while in prison, an important contact with the outside world and a useful part of planning for release. Some agencies are also engaged in providing information and training to staff to broaden their skills repertoire. All these methods can be said to have the broad aims of HIV prevention and improving the treatment of prisoners who are HIV antibody positive, but beyond this they involve different assumptions, commitments and skills, and have different resource implications.

This chapter includes examples of work in prisons in the area of HIV health education. The initiatives included are not meant to be a comprehensive or representative sample, but demonstrate some of the different approaches being taken. The descriptions result from discussions held either with prison staff or staff from community agencies and the comments are not evaluative. The focus is on HIV education but, where substantive reference to the effects of the education or other work on HIV and AIDS has been made, this has also been included.

Saughton Prison, Edinburgh

It may seem strange that a discussion of HIV and AIDS education initiatives in England and Wales should start with a description of a Scottish prison. Saughton has, however, evolved a comprehensive strategy that marks it out as an important example of what can be achieved in the field. It also demonstrates the way that education can be used as a cornerstone of effective HIV/AIDS management in prisons. While there are policy differences between the Scottish Prison Department and that of England and Wales, many of the lessons learned in Saughton are of value to prisons in other parts of Great Britain.

Faced with a high HIV infection rate among injecting drug users in Edinburgh in the mid-1980s, both staff and prisoners feared that they might become infected in prison and also that if they did they might inadvertently infect their families or other sexual partners.

Policy developments in Scottish prisons have been quite different from those in England and Wales, largely because Viral Infectivity Restrictions were never adopted. From an early stage Saughton Prison was able to establish a policy of not segregating prisoners merely on the basis of their HIV antibody status. The aim was to preserve medical confidentiality and to adopt a health and safety policy that treats all body fluid spillages as if they could contain the virus. In late 1988 these decisions were reinforced by the establishment of a multi-disciplinary HIV/AIDS management group. The aims of this group were to ensure the continuance of the integration policy and the strategic development of policies and responses across the prison. Areas highlighted for development were staff training, prisoner education, testing, counselling, confidentiality and services for those who became ill.

Some of the key philosophies behind this approach are that segregation makes the environment more dangerous, increasing complacency with respect to health and safety procedures and fuelling stigmatisation. Furthermore, isolation of prisoners also makes them more difficult to manage. Hence a policy of integrating prisoners with HIV was one that was seen as being of benefit to prisoners, staff and managers. Another element of Saughton's approach was the recognition that uniformed staff could play a role in HIV education and in undertaking basic welfare functions. A third important element was use of the advice and expertise of HIV and drugs services in the local community.

As a starting point the management group commissioned a piece of research to give them a picture of the problem and of the chief anxieties of staff and prisoners with regard to HIV. Subsequently education programmes were devised to provide basic HIV health information for prisoners. These sessions are now run during the induction programme by officers trained in presentation. They are an hour long and they use audio visual materials and discussion. As well as emphasising the risks of drug related behaviour they serve as an opportunity to let the prisoners know about the facilities and policies in Saughton with regard to HIV. Saughton currently has 48 staff trained to undertake this work.

In Edinburgh there is a suggestion that injecting drug use may be decreasing (Greenwood, 1991). In response to this, within the education sessions emphasis is shifting to greater consideration of safer sex. The targeted group is the heterosexual population, with emphasis being placed on transmission outside the prison. A project is currently being explored with the Brook Advisory Service to provide training for prisoners in safer sex counselling for use with their peers in the community. This idea stems from the recognition of the problems faced when telling friends and families about HIV status or about changing sexual practices within a relationship. While these developments are extremely innovative, one possible effect of focusing attention on sex outside the prison could be an avoidance of the issue of sex within the prison.

All staff have received basic information about HIV. In order to keep up to date staff have access to information in a library/resource centre and an occasional newsletter is produced.

Specific skills training is also available to staff. A multi-disciplinary team has been trained in counselling skills. Its services are available to antibody positive prisoners, this being distinct from pre- and post-test counselling which is carried out by hospital staff. Counsellors are trained using materials (Lockley and Williams, 1989) produced by the Scottish Health Education Group (now the Health Education Board for Scotland). The five-day course is run by a prison trainer and an external counselling trainer. Saughton has developed a number of other schemes:

- a fortnightly clinic run by the City Hospital in the prison to undertake health monitoring of prisoners with HIV or AIDS;
- a prisoner support group;
- a poster information campaign;
- a full-time senior social worker who specialises in drugs, HIV and AIDS;
- a buddy scheme organised with Scottish Aids Monitor.

There are also a significant number of plans in development. 'Allermuir', an HIV and AIDS respite care and convalescent facility, has recently been opened inside the prison. Permission has just been granted for a pilot project to be set up, in conjunction with the Community Drug Problem Service and City Hospital, to carry out drug detoxification in the prison. The reduction programme will be up to a maximum of 28 days and will involve psychological support as well.

The HIV/AIDS management group has played a key role in enabling these responses to be developed to some of the issues raised by HIV and AIDS in prison. The committee is now moving its focus to address a drugs brief, the intention being to apply a similar approach to a different problem.

For further information contact The Governor, Saughton Prison, Edinburgh EH1 3LN. Tel: 031-444 2000.

Bristol Prison

The HIV education initiatives at Bristol Prison are probably at the forefront of such work in England and Wales. It is a category B prison for men with a current occupancy of about 360 prisoners, under a third of whom are on remand. Prisoners with HIV are integrated with others on normal location and not barred from taking part in any activities such as work or sport. Bristol's approach involves a comprehensive HIV education programme for staff and prisoners and the development of a confidential counselling service for prisoners. Both the education and counselling are largely carried out and maintained by uniformed staff. This has proved so successful that staff at Bristol now offer training in basic counselling skills to officers from other prisons in the South West.

A mass education programme was undertaken about two years ago when both prisoners and staff were given information about HIV and AIDS. This consisted of a two-hour session incorporating:

- a talk including information about the nature of HIV, transmission routes, safer sex and a demonstration of how to clean a needle and syringe with cold soapy water;
- presentation of the Home Office video *AIDS Inside and Out*;
- discussion of issues arising from the video;
- quiz about HIV and AIDS;
- question-and-answer open forum.

Since then the prison has continued to provide similar education sessions to both new staff and prisoners. For convicted prisoners, for example, sessions are run weekly. Attendance has been compulsory which has had the benefit of ensuring that everyone is included. Recently Bristol has been experimenting with a voluntary approach, in an attempt to respect the differing levels of HIV awareness among prisoners. Planning is currently under way for a pre-release course, the aim being to have it available by the end of September 1991, and it will include an HIV component. It is intended that condoms will be made available to prisoners being released and the local health authority has undertaken to supply the condoms.

The HIV training programme is organised by the HIV education officer, who in addition co-ordinates the counselling service in Bristol Prison and organises HIV courses open to staff from the whole of the Wessex, Wales and West prison areas. The counselling service is advertised on each wing. Prisoners can select whom they wish to approach from a list of prison officers and staff from other disciplines who have received training. Bristol Prison has developed guidelines to ensure that personal information remains confidential. These also require all counsellors to attend training and to keep themselves up to date on HIV.

The course 'Basic Skills in Counselling Techniques' was designed and run in collaboration with the district health authority HIV/AIDS co-ordinator. It lasts four days and covers the basics of HIV and AIDS, pre- and post-test counselling, support, talking to people about their worries and, most important, confidentiality.

The model used at Bristol evolved and grew in response to identified needs. Education eased the introduction of an integration policy within the prison and also highlighted the need for personal support for staff and prisoners, and in response to this a counselling service was developed. These changes meant that Bristol was acting differently from the other prisons in the area, which had implications for the treatment of HIV antibody positive prisoners who might move to prisons operating a segregation policy. Negotiation was undertaken with the then regional training department to offer the courses to other prisons.

Bristol Prison has had a significant impact on the policy and practice of other prisons in the south west of England. For instance, Winchester, Dorchester and Portland are now carrying out HIV education for prisoners and have adopted a counselling service. Gloucester is starting a programme of officer training and a network of contacts between prison staff is developing. This means that Bristol can hand on the names of counsellors in some other prisons to transferring prisoners who may decide to use this information. A great strength of the Bristol model has been the ability to work realistically but effectively within the constraints set by the availability of time, staff and cash.

The process did not happen in a vacuum. It was informed by other developments in the field such as those at Saughton Prison in Edinburgh and use was made of the Prison Department educational materials. The work has considerable support from the Governor and Bristol Prison's management. An HIV/AIDS working party was established to devise the integration policy and it was recognised that in order to effect these changes negotiation needed to be carried out with all levels of staff. Finally, community-based organisations have also been called upon to offer valuable resources such as joint training, information and assisting prison staff in keeping up to date with developments in the HIV field.

For further information contact Geoff Marlow, HIV Education Officer, Bristol Prison, Cambridge Road, Bristol BS7 8PS. Tel: 0272 426661.

Grendon Prison

Grendon is located near Aylesbury and has accommodation for about 200 men serving medium- and long-term sentences. Each wing operates as a therapeutic community which makes Grendon unique within the prison system of England and Wales. It is a relatively small prison and there is usually a long waiting list of people seeking to transfer there. Prisoners are expected to work in addition to participating actively in the therapy groups. One of the aims of these groups is to give people some insight into their offences which may help them not to re-offend. Newly trained officers assigned to Grendon often discover skills in group work that they were unaware of previously. Grendon has a reputation for maintaining a high level of trust and co-operation between staff and prisoners, which is important for the therapeutic model and can also provide a good setting in which to educate people about HIV and AIDS.

At Grendon it was decided not to enforce the Viral Infectivity Restrictions when they were introduced by the Prison Department in 1985. There was, however, an awareness of the need to educate staff and prisoners about HIV and AIDS. In addition there was a recognition of the importance of observing appropriate health, hygiene and safety standards.

In the early stages several officers sought information about HIV on their own initiative and made it available to prisoners and staff on an informal basis. Later some officers attended a training course in the south west region – a local initiative set up by Bristol Prison and the local health education department (described elsewhere in this chapter). This served to supplement existing knowledge and to provide an opportunity to explore ways in which HIV education and advice could be delivered to prisoners.

At present when people arrive at Grendon they are placed in the assessment unit for several months to see which wing will provide the most appropriate form of therapy. A one-and-a-half- to two-hour session on HIV/AIDS is held in this unit usually once every six weeks. There is no need for greater frequency because of the low turnover of prisoners and the length of the assessment period. A prison officer introduces the session, shows the prison video *AIDS Inside and Out*, and then leads a general discussion for about an hour on questions raised by the video. Although the sessions are primarily for prisoners, prison staff are welcome to attend and often take part in the discussion. Some prisoners still in the assessment unit may choose to attend a repeat session to review their knowledge or ask questions which they have thought of since the first session.

The use of drugs is a sensitive issue at Grendon. It is considered that the illicit use of drugs may diminish the benefits that prisoners can gain in the therapy groups. However, staff recognise that people may still decide to take drugs in and out of Grendon and have therefore introduced some basic risk reduction information relating to HIV transmission and drug use. Part of this is a demonstration on how to clean a syringe and needle. Diluted washing up liquid is suggested as a cleaning agent as bleach is not freely available to prisoners.

Any prisoner who is considering having an HIV antibody test may speak to the prison medical officer who either counsels him or refers him to a prison officer trained in pre-test counselling. Tests are carried out by a local doctor from a genito-urinary medicine clinic who visits the prison, and results are recorded on the prisoner's medical record.

General information about HIV and AIDS is made available to staff and prisoners by the trained officers. Two publications are described as being particularly useful: *Smack in the Eye*, produced by the Lifeline Project, Manchester, and the *Mainliners Newsletter*.

Grendon has developed strong working relationships with local statutory and voluntary organisations in the HIV and AIDS field. An example of this is the HIV component of a pre-release course run jointly by Grendon staff and an HIV trainer from Aylesbury Vale Health Authority at the nearby Spring Hill Prison.

Separate training for staff has been arranged periodically and is held in facilities provided by the training department. Although HIV and AIDS may not have as high a profile as at Saughton or Bristol prisons, the level of education and support for prisoners and staff dovetails neatly with the philosophy of the regime.

For further information contact Robert Shepherd, Hospital Principal Officer, Grendon Prison, Grendon Underwood, Aylesbury, Buckinghamshire HP18 0TL. Tel: 0296 770301 ext 387.

Hollesley Bay Young Offender Institution

In 1989 a joint initiative between the Suffolk Probation Service and the East Anglian Regional Health Authority resulted in the appointment of three full-time probation service employed health co-ordinators to cover the prisons within the region. These posts are totally funded by the health authority.

Their main role is to educate prisoners and staff about HIV and AIDS and to liaise with other disciplines within the institution involved in addressing drug problems and health and social issues with prisoners. In addition they provide counselling (they are trained HIV/AIDS counsellors), develop educational resources, provide up-to-date information, and liaise with external statutory and voluntary agencies in the HIV/AIDS field. These posts are not necessarily filled by probation officers, in fact the co-ordinator at Hollesley Bay has a nursing background.

Hollesley Bay is a young offender institution for 500 17–21 year old males, divided into two parts – open and secure. The role of the probation health co-ordinator was approved by a multi-disciplinary working party and the Governor. An initial discussion document noted that a high proportion of young offenders had a history of drug use and some had little knowledge of high-risk behaviour relating to the transmission of HIV.

Health education concerning HIV, AIDS and drugs is provided for staff and prisoners in several ways. For prisoners the aim is that all young people attend a one-and-a-half hour session during their first week which is led by the probation health co-ordinator and a teacher from the education department. There are plans to involve trained prison officers in the delivery of this education programme. Sessions are held in both the open and secure sections of the institution.

AIDS Inside and Out is shown and the leaflet which accompanies it is distributed. There are opportunities in the sessions for discussion and to respond to specific questions and issues which the video may raise.

A ten-week drug course, operating one day a week, is offered to prisoners with contributions from the probation health co-ordinator, the prison consultant psychiatrist, the local community drug team, Alcoholics Anonymous and Narcotics Anonymous. A weekly drug group is also available for young prisoners and is run in conjunction with prison officers. Individual counselling is offered by the probation health co-ordinator, prison officers from the personal officer scheme and outside agencies. Before release prisoners have the opportunity to attend further courses on issues relating to their return to the community which may include drug misuse and high-risk behaviour relating to the transmission of HIV.

A resource pack produced by the probation department is offered to all prisoners leaving the institution whether it be on permanent release, home leave or pre-parole leave. This pack includes condoms, a leaflet about safer sex and information about organisations which offer counselling, information and support. The issuing of the resource pack is supported by Dr Rosemary Wool, the Director of the Prison Medical Service.

Training for staff has focused on the personal officer scheme, which has highlighted further training needs, including HIV, AIDS and substance misuse. A six-week course, one day a week, facilitated by Relate, has been attended by 18 staff, many of whom have expressed an interest in further training in the HIV/AIDS and substance misuse field. Sixty-eight prison staff have attended internal drugs awareness days which were led jointly by staff from the community drug team, Suffolk Community Alcohol Service and the local health promotion unit. In addition to this some officers have attended courses run by the local health authority on HIV and AIDS.

For further information contact Barbara Marsh, Probation Health Co-ordinator, Hollesley Bay, Woodbridge, Suffolk IP12 3JS. Tel 0394 411741.

Holloway Prison

Holloway is the largest prison for women in England and Wales. It is a local prison with both a remand and convicted population and is situated in central London.

HIV and AIDS awareness education for prisoners occurs within several different locations in the prison. The main areas involved are the activities centre, the education department and the medical unit.

The activities centre organises three courses: induction, pre-release, and a six-week drug and alcohol rehabilitation course. These courses are run by discipline staff with outside agencies being used to facilitate the HIV and AIDS awareness and harm minimisation sessions within them. For example, Central London Action on Street Health (CLASH) run a session on induction, Healthy Options Team (HOT) a session on pre-release. A typical format is to show the Home office video *AIDS Inside and Out* and facilitate a discussion, followed by exercises or a quiz.

The drug and alcohol rehabilitation course provides a further opportunity to look at issues raised by HIV, AIDS and drug use. The course incorporates a harm minimisation approach, using the expertise of a number of outside agencies. Examples of the groups involved include Positively Women, The Angel Project, Mainliners, Terrence Higgins Trust, The Samaritans and CLASH. The course also looks at alternative approaches to health and relaxation such as reflexology, massage and acupuncture. About 14 women usually attend the course. It is advertised in the prison but most women hear of it by word of mouth and then apply for an assessment interview.

Prison officers do not attend the sessions which address HIV awareness and harm minimisation as it is felt that this may inhibit discussion of risky behaviour. A new course planned for next January is entitled the Personal Empowerment Project. The steering committee is multi-disciplinary and also includes one serving prisoner and two Holloway ex-prisoners. HIV and AIDS awareness groups are also held in the education department and the medical unit.

AIDS Inside and Out is used extensively as an educational tool though there are reservations about how adequately it addresses the concerns or needs of women. This criticism is based on both its content and style. Issues that could be included, or covered better, are pregnancy, childbirth and children in relation to HIV or AIDS, women on the street, lesbianism, assertiveness and a wider perspective on safer sex.

A regular Holloway liaison meeting is held, attended by prison staff (mainly discipline, probation and psychology) and any of the outside agencies involved in the HIV health education process. This group provides an opportunity for staff from different projects and from the prison to meet, discuss problems that might arise, provide support and generate new ideas.

It is not known what proportion of the prisoners actually attend at least one basic HIV awareness session. Blackburn (1991) has calculated that only 22.2 per cent of all admissions attended induction in January 1991. Pre-release courses are a fortnight long and open to 12 women at a time. Even with the other initiatives in the prison it is unlikely that all prisoners are receiving basic information.

Pre-test counselling is available from the 'special clinic' run by the medical unit. Counselling can also be arranged from the psychology or probation departments, but it can take up to two weeks from request to interview. The hospital provides treatment for prisoners with drug use problems, including a 7–10 day methadone reduction programme where appropriate.

On a final note, the prison has been trying out different ways of making condoms freely and anonymously available to prisoners on temporary release, home leave or discharge. Unfortunately, it has not proved easy to find an acceptable way of reaching only the target population, preserving anonymity and getting someone to pay the condom bill.

For further information contact Deborah Blackburn, Activities Centre, Holloway Prison, Parkhurst Road, London N7 0NU. Tel: 071-607 6747.

West Midlands Regional Health Authority

So far the descriptions have covered work from within prisons. The following accounts offer a contrast. The first is the perspective of a Senior Health Promotion Officer (SHPO), Pat McKenzie from mid-Staffordshire, developing a collaborative working relationship with six prisons within Staffordshire.

The Senior Health Promotion Officer (HIV/AIDS with Offenders) is a new post created in November 1990 and is probably unique in this country. The role of the post is to raise awareness about HIV and AIDS through education and training of staff and prisoners in four young offender institutions: Brinsford, Drake Hall, Werrington and Swinfen Hall, and two prisons: Featherstone and Stafford.

Pat McKenzie made initial approaches to the prison education departments to find out what education and training had been done already around HIV and AIDS, and to make contact with people. The District Health Promotion Officer (DHPO) had previously developed contacts with prison education officers which resulted in visits to prisons to offer information and training materials on general health issues – not specifically about HIV and AIDS. It was felt that there was a need for specific training on HIV and AIDS.

Following these initial contacts, Pat McKenzie was invited to lead joint sessions with teachers about HIV, AIDS and drugs awareness on a variety of courses offered to prisoners in different prisons. The input on the courses was evaluated by giving the teacher, who sat in on the sessions, a questionnaire to complete. This helped Pat to make improvements in the running of the sessions. Stafford and Drake Hall prisons have been involved in particularly interesting developments in this field. Pat McKenzie was invited to organise a four-day HIV and AIDS training course for staff at Stafford Prison with an HIV education officer from Bristol Prison. Some of the officers who attended expressed an interest in acting as prison officer counsellors to offer support and advice to prisoners worried about issues relating to HIV and AIDS.

Stafford was considering the removal of Viral Infectivity Restrictions (VIR) but more information was needed about how this could best be done before a final decision was made. Several staff visited Bristol and Saughton Prisons where VIR is not used. The four-day course on HIV and AIDS helped to increase awareness that VIR was not necessary. The SHPO was subsequently invited to become a member of the HIV/AIDS Management Committee. The responsibilities of the committee were to develop an HIV/AIDS policy for Stafford and to oversee the removal of VIR. The other members of the committee included a governor grade, principal officer (training), senior probation officer, chaplain, education officer, prison officer (who represents the prison officer counsellors), a representative of the Prison Officers Association, and the HIV co-ordinator from the local social services department.

At the time of writing (August 1991) VIR has not yet been removed. Until it is, a VIR group for prisoners continues to meet to support those who are segregated under VIR and may feel isolated. Pat McKenzie helps in the running of this group.

Pat organised HIV and AIDS awareness courses for staff and offered support, information and advice to prison staff trainers who wanted to present HIV and AIDS awareness sessions to their colleagues. She sat in on two presentations to see what areas needed further work. As a result 'training the trainers' groups were organised to formulate aims and objectives and to develop methods of evaluating them. Methods of learning were discussed further and staff practised their presentations. These were recorded on video to enable participants to see themselves and make any changes they felt necessary to improve the quality of their presentations. The long-term plan at Stafford is that prison staff will adapt the education package for groups of prisoners. The size of these has yet to be determined but the SHPO would prefer a maximum of 15 to allow as much participation as possible.

At Drake Hall, a women's prison and young offender institution, a six-to eight-week course is available to prisoners covering subjects including drugs, HIV and AIDS, employment, social skills, etc. Pat McKenzie was invited to lead two sessions on HIV and AIDS awareness on an eight-week course and also to provide input to a drug users' group run by prison officers as part of a pre-release course. She has also been involved in leading sessions with a teacher on other courses within the prison. These are evaluated as described earlier.

There are many issues relating to HIV and AIDS which concern women specifically such as pregnancy, child care and sexual assault which are addressed on these courses. Pat McKenzie has led discussion groups with women awaiting deportation which have highlighted some difficult and sensitive issues about HIV, AIDS and racism.

There are plans to run a three-day multi-disciplinary training course for staff on HIV and AIDS, drugs, listening skills and groupwork.

In addition to direct work with prisoners, education departments and prison officers, Pat McKenzie has been responsible for liaising with local voluntary and statutory organisations. She has developed contacts with Body Positive and drug agencies within the county which provide specialist counselling to prisoners on issues relating to HIV, AIDS and drugs.

Several points which have been particularly helpful in developing Pat's work in the prisons include:

- previous contacts – prison staff understood the role of health promotion officers;
- finding out what makes prisons 'tick' – routines, departmental structures, rules, etc.;
- the service offered to the prison is free;
- getting to know prison staff of different grades and departments on a personal level.

In contrast a significant hindrance was the denial to varying degrees that HIV and AIDS created a problem in prisons. Pat McKenzie describes herself primarily as an 'enabler'. She recognises that many prison staff have latent talents in group and communication skills and simply need an opportunity to discover and use them. Some may choose to use them in HIV education in prison, others will not.

For further information contact Patricia McKenzie, Senior Health Promotion Officer, First Community Health, Mellor House, Corporation Street, Stafford ST16 3SR Tel: 0785 222888 ext 5229.

Leicestershire HIV/AIDS and Drugs Prison Project

In order to ensure that adequate HIV and drug services are available to the five prisons in the county, Leicestershire probation service and Leicester Community Drug Services have set up a joint venture. The Department of Health have funded the secondment of a probation officer to the Leicester Action for Youth Trust's Drugs Advice Centre for three years from April 1990.

At the time of writing the project is still at a relatively early stage. The difficulty of obtaining a continuing commitment of time and resources from the prisons on the issue of HIV has at times made progress frustratingly slow for the worker involved. She has managed to train probation officers seconded to all five Leicestershire establishments in one-day HIV awareness courses. Both Glen Parva Young Offender Institution and Gartree Prison (dispersal) have multi-disciplinary HIV/AIDS working groups on which the project worker sits. At Glen Parva a three-day HIV awareness course was held for staff from a range of disciplines. This is to be followed in the near future by a further four-day HIV awareness course designed once more for a multi-disciplinary group. The course will include a risk assessment component to train staff to determine whether someone expressing concern over possible exposure to HIV has any grounds for anxiety. If it seems that the individual has placed himself at risk and is asking for a blood test he will be referred to a counsellor for pre-test counselling.

In her first annual report the project worker, Sue Whitlock, reflects on a number of lessons to be learnt from the first year of the project. These include:

- the need to achieve a high personal profile within the prisons by means of frequent visits, targeted communication and membership of working groups;
- the advantage of encouraging a multi-disciplinary approach to HIV, AIDS and drugs;
- the importance of obtaining the support of the overall governor of the

prison rather than relying on contacts at the governor IV and V level. These governors have specific areas of responsibility, and may find it difficult to marshal the necessary resources alone. They also seem to move posts frequently;

● the advantage of assessing staff training needs thoroughly. It is important to be clear what staff require and a formal training needs analysis using an interview schedule is an effective way of achieving this.

Future plans for the Leicestershire project include a conference for staff from the Leicestershire prisons and outside organisations working with them, the production of a newsletter, the formation of a support group for those involved in the prison HIV working groups in the county, and further training including the training of trainers within the prisons.

For further information contact Sue Whitlock, Project Worker, Drug Advice Centre, Paget House, 2 West Street, Leicester LE1 6XP. Tel: 0533 470200.

Prison Brokerage Scheme

The Prison Brokerage Scheme was initiated by the National AIDS Trust (NAT) to facilitate work in prisons by community-based organisations. It is part of the National AIDS and Prisons Consortium Project, which is a collaboration between NAT, the National Association for the Care and Resettlement of Offenders, the Parole Release Scheme and the Terrence Higgins Trust. The initial aim was for a 'broker' to be employed to cover each of the four administrative regions the Prison Department then used. The northern broker, Di Robertson, was appointed in November 1990 with two years' funding from the Home Office Drugs Branch to cover the area from Liverpool in the west to South Yorkshire in the east and north to the Scottish border. Unlike the south east brokerage, which was the first and is based at the Parole Release Scheme agency, the northern broker operates independently of any agency, though she uses office space at Body Positive North East.

For Di Robertson brokerage involves mediating between people working in prisons and those working in outside agencies in relation to HIV, and maximising the benefits of contact. Of course, many community-based drug and HIV agencies have been working closely with prisons for some time. In order to establish what was already happening when she started work on the brokerage, Di Robertson wrote about 300 letters to agencies in the north working in the HIV and drug fields to ask what prison work was under way. About a third responded and she organised localised meetings to gain a clearer picture and assess what more could be done. From these local meetings a number of 'outsider' groups have emerged which meet on a regular basis. These provide much needed support for workers who may receive little understanding from their own agencies about the stresses of prison work. They also enable the workers themselves to use their resources effectively, avoiding duplication of effort and identifying specific needs within their local area. Another important facet of the work has been highlighting HIV and arranging specific training around the issue for other agencies offering general advice services in prisons such as the Samaritans and Citizens Advice Bureaux.

Introducing the brokerage scheme to the prisons in the northern area has proved more difficult. Peter Done of the Directorate of the Prison Medical Service wrote to all managing medical officers with copies to all governors in the region to convey the message that the brokerage scheme enjoyed DPMS support. Di Robertson then wrote an introductory letter to all managing medical officers asking basic questions in order to gain a general picture of HIV and drug service provision and to identify any gaps.

The response from prisons has been very patchy. Many of the prisons in the area have hardly had any dealings with HIV so far, and prevalence is also low in many communities in the area. For some prisons it does not appear to be a major issue yet. It also appears that in some prisons the medical staff are unaware of drug or HIV agencies who provide a regular service to the prison. These agencies may have decided not to go through the medical staff but to gain access via the probation or education departments or the pre-release course.

These introductory letters have been followed by visits from Di Robertson which allow better assessment of any need for services or training. Although the provision of training is not the immediate responsibility of the broker, Di has been involved in running two one-day HIV awareness courses for management at Manchester Prison and will take part in a similar venture at Leeds Prison in the autumn. She is also organising training for a small number of officers at the Durham prisons in collaboration with Durham's HIV Prevention Co-ordinator and Body

Positive County Durham. Other agencies in the northern region are involved increasingly in offering training on HIV and drugs to staff from the prisons in which they work.

To date only Manchester and Askham Grange Prisons in the northern region have convened multi-disciplinary HIV/AIDS committees. As the number doing so inevitably increases, the role of the broker is likely to become ever more crucial in maintaining HIV prevention as a high priority in the prisons, and in ensuring the best possible contact with, and distribution of, the valuable resources of community-based organisations in the prisons.

For further information contact Di Robertson, c/o Body Positive North East, MEA House, Ellison Place, Newcastle on Tyne NE1 8XS. Tel: 091-232 2855.

South-east regional broker: Mike Trace, Parole Release Scheme, 93 Fortess Road, London NW5 1AG. Tel: 071-267 4446.

Midlands regional broker: Sally Perkins, c/o NACRO, 107 Soho Hill, Birmingham B19 1AY. Tel: 021-554 2266.

Chapter 6

Working Together –
Prisons and the Community

One of the most welcome proposals contained in the Woolf Report following the prison disturbances of 1990 was the idea of community prisons. The practice of allocating prisoners to gaols distant from their home area has the effect not only of damaging or destroying relationships with family and friends, it also creates problems for community-based agencies who should ideally be able to make links with people while they are in custody and continue to offer a service after release. The notion of a community prison implies that prisoners will remain closer to their home communities and also that the prison will participate as part of that community.

Over the past decade prisons have become increasingly accessible to outside organisations wishing to provide services to individual prisoners or to particular groups such as those with alcohol problems or on pre-release courses. The role of community-based drug agencies is specifically mentioned in the recent guidance on the throughcare of drug users and in the accompanying manual *Caring for Drug Users* (Prison Department, 1991). The Woolf Report also stresses the importance of local drug and HIV agencies in providing services for prisoners (see Appendix 3), and this is reiterated in the Government White Paper *Custody Care and Justice* (1991). However, the relationship between prisons and 'outsiders' has not always been easy. Provision of services to prisons is often patchy and under-resourced and co-ordination of activities within prisons woefully inadequate. If Woolf's vision of the community prison is to be translated into reality, a more methodical approach to the co-ordination of links between a prison and community-based organisations must be adopted.

Of course, there have been cases where outside organisations have acted unprofessionally, and some prisons in turn have been obstructive and reluctant to welcome 'outsiders'. But many of the difficulties that arise do so simply because of differences in expectations and misunderstandings.

Although some guidance has been available to outsiders, prisons themselves have not previously been given any specific information on working with community agencies. This chapter is divided into two sections to provide information and useful suggestions. It is designed to be applicable both in situations where the outside agency is working with prisoners directly as well as where the main focus is staff training. The appendices which follow are designed to facilitate initial contacts. All the prisons in England and Wales are listed and matched with their regional and district health authorities and prison areas, and national organisations dealing with HIV, drugs and prisons are included.

Working with Prisons – a Guide for Community-based Agencies

For workers in community-based agencies, prison work can be both attractive and rewarding. Some prisoners use their time in prison to take stock and may be amenable to change. Almost all appreciate contact with the outside world and a diversion from the usual routine. So whether an outside service offers group or individual work there is likely to be a positive response from prisoners. But how does one get to that stage?

Preparing for Prison Work

Embarking on prison work can be a major commitment for an agency with other functions to fulfil, and there are a number of issues which may usefully be considered before even starting the process of gaining access. Perhaps the most fundamental is *why prison work is being considered*. It may be that the agency has a number of clients in one particular prison, or that the prison itself falls within the agency's catchment area. Perhaps the agency wants to help the prison improve the service to a particular client group by offering inmate education or staff training. Following on from this is the question of *what service is being offered and how much time the agency can devote to it*. Providing a regular service to a prison is extremely time-consuming since it often involves travelling, waiting (getting from the gate to wherever work is to take place can take a while), and liaison with members of prison staff as well as the actual time in the group or counselling. Contact with prisoners may also have implications for the role of the agency in the community. Is the intention simply to provide a service to people while they are in prison or will this extend to diversion from custody schemes for people on remand, through expectations or even conditions of attendance linked to probation orders for drug and alcohol users, for example? How does the agency see its role in terms of aftercare and parole? *Reliability* is extremely important both from the point of view of the prisoner(s) involved and in terms of the reputation of the agency. In fact, unreliability on the part of one agency can even affect the prospects of workers from completely different organisations receiving a positive response from the prison. Because the need to be able to fulfil commitments to the prison is so strong it is important that the *effect prison work will have on the resources available for the other work of the agency is properly considered. It is important that the aims of prison work are clear, the boundaries of any commitment well defined, and the long-term strategy for such work within the agency properly thought out before work starts.*

Making Contact

Gaining access to a prison often seems the most formidable initial task. How contact is initiated can have an important effect on what happens afterwards.

There is no guaranteed route since in every prison the allocation of tasks seems slightly different. For example, in some prisons groups for drug users are run by the psychology or probation departments. In others drug use is covered almost exclusively by a prison officer specialising in that area or on the pre-release course. But in some prisons virtually no services are available for drug users and no general information on drug use provided at all. Likewise with HIV education – it may be the preserve of the hospital, staff running pre-release or induction courses, education department, probation department, specified discipline staff, another outside agency or simply not be taking place. Moreover, liaison and communications between departments in prisons are not always good, so that one department may be unaware of the work already going on elsewhere in the prison, or have a negative view of it.

If a good contact point has been suggested by someone who is in a position to know, of course it is sensible to make use of it. Otherwise *a letter to the prison governor* outlining any proposal may be useful since it can be discussed at the governor's daily meeting attended by all senior managers within the prison and will be passed on to the most appropriate department.

While initial contact is being established it is important to *find out what else is happening in the prison* with regard to the type of work proposed. Other local agencies may already be providing services to the prison and it is obviously important to avoid duplication and competition. If this is the case they may be able to highlight any deficiencies in existing service provision and suggest useful contact points in the prison.

At some prisons workers from community-based agencies have formed prison workers groups which meet regularly to discuss issues of common interest, provide mutual support and communicate with the governor as a group about any shared difficulties.

Once contact has been made it may be a good idea to ask *if the prospective prison worker can spend some time with members of various departments in the institution.* This not only creates an opportunity to find out if any parallel work is already under way, but also affords valuable insight into the way the prison operates. It is also a good idea for any *interested prison staff to be offered the opportunity to visit the agency concerned* so that they may put the service provided at the prison into its community-based context.

Negotiation of work to be undertaken in a prison can be complex and lengthy. Because of shift systems the membership of committees can vary from one meeting to another. To avoid covering the same ground time after time it is advisable to *ensure that meetings are minuted* (not necessarily by the outside agency!) and that any proposals are presented in writing. It may prove useful to *aim at negotiating some form of contract with the prison* about the type of service to be offered, expectations in terms of confidentiality, access, support from the prison (availability of rooms, officers to escort, etc.), and the structure for liaison and review.

Under the new funding arrangements for prisons it is now possible for some financial support to be made available to outside organisations providing regular services to individual institutions. Since budget forecasts have to be prepared each financial year it may be that funds are not immediately available when work commences, but it is worth asking about support for the future either at the negotiating stage or when work has become established.

While some prisons are not so welcoming, others are very keen to work with outsiders and may generate all sorts of ideas as to what could be done. When negotiating it is worth considering any options suggested by the prison, but it is important not to be seduced into over-committing the agency because of the enthusiasm of members of the prison staff. Taking on too much can lead to disappointment and disillusion on all sides.

The way in which prisoners will reach your service and the implications of this for them must be carefully considered at this stage. How will they be referred? Will the service be generally advertised and open to all? How will prisoners get from where they are to where the service is being offered? Will their contact with the agency automatically create confidentiality problems (i.e. by identifying those who may have concerns about HIV or drugs, for example)? If so, what effect will identification have on prisoners (for example, will expressing concern about a drug problem lead to extra searches of the prisoner's cell and person)? How will the agency be identified at the prison gate where identification must be shown? Will the worker become known as 'the AIDS lady' or 'the drugs man'? There are no easy answers to these dilemmas and the best solution varies from prison to prison. It is vital to be aware that in most prisons prisoners have no freedom of movement. They have to be escorted from place to place by officers and their movements have to be accounted for.

Working with Prisoners

Once the process of negotiation is complete and work finally starts it can be extremely intense and absorbing. *Many prisoners have relatively little contact with the outside world, an enormous amount of time to think and are extremely bored.* Workers involved with individual prisoners often find the experience both rewarding and highly pressurised. *It is essential to bear in mind the amount of time prisoners spend alone*, since an upsetting counselling session with insufficient 'resolution' time, or a confrontational group, can have a devastating impact. In some prisons there is no evening recreation period so an afternoon session may be followed by a meal, and then the prisoner could be locked up until the next morning with no escape or diversion from any distressing emotions aroused during counselling or groupwork.

Confidentiality is an even more important issue in groupwork conducted in a prison than outside. Participants can easily become carried away by being able to talk in a way not normally possible in a prison and may say more than they intend. An unscrupulous group member could make life difficult as a result. This should be taken into account when groupwork programmes are being organised and prisoners should perhaps be reminded of the environment they are in.

Maintaining an effective professional relationship can prove difficult for similar reasons. It is easy for someone in prison to become emotionally dependent on an outside contact who clearly cares and is interested in the prisoner's welfare. It is sometimes difficult for the prisoner to perceive the worker as part of an agency if contact always takes the form of one-to-one contact in the prison visits room. Again there are no simple answers, but it is advisable to *stick to and reiterate the boundaries of contact established at the outset* and to reinforce the fact that this is part of the agency's prison work to forestall any mis-understandings.

Prisoners may sometimes put pressure on workers to break the rules, particularly in relation to bringing in money, drugs, etc. It is important that those involved in prison work from the outside are aware of the rules; a useful source of information for this and general background on the prison routine is provided by the Prisoners' Information Pack available from the Prison Reform Trust. If workers from community-based agencies do break the rules (by bringing in illicit items, for example) they must be aware that the penalties are high. Not only do they risk criminal prosecution, but the prisoner is also likely to be disciplined and, if found guilty, may lose remission and possibly the prospect of parole. Individuals may decide to run personal risks, but it is important to realise that even *a simple and small-scale breach of the rules will wreck other prison work by that agency and will jeopardise the efforts of other outside agencies at that prison and probably many others besides.* Nothing travels faster than bad news.

Maintaining a professional image in the prison is important in terms of the way the work of the agency is valued by the prison, which can affect the time and space allowed to it and referrals. *It is a good idea to get an ID card* made up to ease access. The prison may decide to 'vet' potential prison workers by checking on criminal records. This means basic information is usually required about potential prison workers. Prison governors receive guidance from the Prison Service that workers who have been convicted in the past should not necessarily be refused access. Each case is considered on its merits and factors such as the length of time since conviction, the nature of the offence, the nature of work proposed at the prison, the security category of the prison, and the level of supervision to be provided by prison staff are all taken into account in reaching a decision. *Dressing appropriately* also contributes to the way a worker is regarded. While it may feel satisfying to make a statement through personal appearance, in a prison those who will be made most aware of the reaction are the prisoners/clients after the worker has left.

Because prisoners have very restricted possibilities when it comes to communicating with the outside world, workers providing services will often be asked if they can help by passing on messages, helping to find employment, etc. *It is particularly important to keep any promises made* in this situation and not to suggest possibilities which are unlikely to come to fruition. 'I don't know if I can do much about accommodation. If I hear of anything I'll let you know' might sound like an idle expression of benevolent intent. To a prisoner desperate for somewhere to live, going over what was said during an interview time and time again it may be transformed into 'X is going to look out for accommodation' and then 'X is going to find me accommodation'.

When acting on behalf of a prisoner it is as well to keep in contact with other agencies in touch with the same person (e.g. the probation service) to make sure that no unnecessary duplication is taking place. Because outside workers often don't seem to do what they say they will, prisoners quite often hedge their bets by asking several people to do the same thing. This sometimes leads to individuals being unfairly described as 'manipulative'. It may be that most sensible people given such limited means of communication and influence over their own lives would develop such skills as a means of survival.

Reliability in terms of attending the prison when appointments have been made has already been mentioned. *If a worker is unable to keep a prison appointment it is very important* not simply to inform the switchboard or gate, but *to make sure that the prisoners due to be seen are also told beforehand.* This may be achieved by asking the probation officer/psychologist/ teacher or other contact point to let them know. Alternatively, it may be useful to have a record of each of the client/prisoner's locations within the prison (wing or unit) and ask staff on duty there to pass messages to the prisoners concerned. Of course, prisoners may be unable to get messages to outside workers if they are not going to keep appointments (if, for example, a prisoner is transferred to another prison at short notice). *It may be advisable to phone the prison on the morning of the visit or session to check*, if there is any prospect of the prisoner/client being moved or if the worker has to travel some distance.

The routine in most prisons means that generally work with prisoners can take place for about two hours in the morning (9.30–11.30) and about the same in the afternoon (1.30–3.30). This varies from one prison to another but there is normally a period of around two hours in the middle of the day when prisoners are not available while they and then the prison staff have lunch. Spending a whole day at a prison can involve quite a lot of time spent waiting.

Unfortunately, both prisoners and outside workers sometimes feel they have grounds for complaint about the way they have been treated, so it is important to be aware of how to deal with such difficulties. Prisoners have a grievance procedure open to them but if this does not seem to be achieving anything an outside worker could write to the Governor or Chairman of the Board of Visitors. If the prisoner still feels aggrieved it may be worth putting him/her in touch with the Prisoners' Advice and Legal Service, 708 Holloway Road, London N19 3NL, or the Prison Reform Trust, 59 Caledonian Road, London N1 9BU. It is important to maintain an awareness of the role of the agency and, having referred the prisoner on, not to jeopardise the other work the agency is involved in at the prison. Outside workers wishing to complain on their own behalf should go first to the main point of contact, then to the Governor.

Adequate supervision and support are of crucial importance to workers involved in prison work. Many people find visiting a prison a distressing experience in itself. This is compounded by the difficulties faced by prisoners who are rendered helpless by virtue of their imprisonment. The emotional pressure can be intense and supervisors need to be sufficiently skilled to deal with it. Difficulties sometimes arise for workers who are supervised by people with no knowledge or experience of prisons. In such situations it may be advisable to consider finding additional support through a local prison workers' group. These may be based around an area or focused on one prison. Alternatively it may be possible to form links with a local probation team which might employ a specialist prison worker or someone who specialises in alcohol or drugs, for example, but who will inevitably be experienced in working with prisoners.

Working with Community-based Agencies – a Guide for Prisons

Prisons have opened their doors to increasing numbers of people working for outside agencies over the last decade. But the scale of such involvement could be far greater if it were made a little easier and less daunting for community-based agencies to make initial contact and if liaison thereafter was improved. In many areas there are outsiders who are keen to offer an expert service to prisons, often at no cost, and generally they have no choice but to do so on the prison's terms.

Although it may seem strange to those working in a prison every day *the prospect of making the first contact can prove daunting to an outside worker.* Many are unsure who to contact initially and have no idea of the complicated staffing structure of a prison. The language too can prove baffling, so to be told 'No, you need to talk to the Head of Inmate Activities' for example, can be distinctly unhelpful. It is easy, when working in an enclosed and structured environment, to forget just how strange it can be to an outsider.

Preparing to Work with Outside Agencies

Although prisons sometimes ask local agencies for assistance it seems that more often the approach comes from the community-based organisation. It would be a refreshing change if prisons did request the attention of external agencies a little more often. *In order to locate services* where no existing contacts exist, *national organisations often keep details of local agencies and they can easily be approached.* For example, the Standing Conference on Drug Abuse maintains local lists of drug agencies, the *National AIDS Manual* contains a comprehensive directory of HIV-related services. A useful starting point for HIV services may be the District HIV Prevention Co-ordinator or DHPC (see Appendix 5, part 1). People in prison are one of the target groups for prevention defined for DHPCs by the Department of Health, and the Prison Medical Directorate has recently written to all institutions to encourage contact. DHPCs can facilitate contact with local HIV agencies. The three regional prison brokers (see Chapter 5) may also be able to help. The next task a prison is faced with after contact has been established is deciding whether the organisation is bona fide, whether the service offered is appropriate and what the resource implications will be.

The overwhelming majority of organisations approaching prisons with a view to offering services are likely to be doing so with the best of motives and as a way of extending their existing service provision. Unfortunately, the idea of working with prisons also attracts a few people who want to use prisoners to try out dubious and unorthodox approaches to various problems or who are motivated at least in part by voyeurism. If in doubt it may be advisable to *check the reputation of an agency with other existing contacts in the field or with one of the national organisations.* Voluntary agencies all publish annual reports and should be able to provide copies on request. In order to obtain a clear picture of the philosophy and context of work offered it may be useful for a member of the prison staff to visit the agency. This sounds obvious, but there is often an assumption that all contact will occur on prison territory.

The type of service offered and resource implications for the prison need to be clearly negotiated at the outset. Though this may be undertaken by an individual (probation officer, psychologist, Head of Inmate Activities), it may be useful to arrange at least one meeting with any others likely to be affected so that everyone is fully informed about what is happening. If agreement is required before work can proceed it may be worth asking the agency to produce a written proposal and to negotiate a contract with them clarifying expectations and responsibilities on all sides. If it is simply a matter of letting others know what is happening, holding a seminar to which representatives of relevant departments are invited may prove useful. In any event it may be valuable to decide at the outset how the progress of work undertaken will be reviewed to ensure that any difficulties on the part of either the prison or the agency can be resolved and that the continuing relevance of the service offered can be assessed.

Working with Outsiders

For co-operation with outside agencies to work well it is important that good and trusting relationships are established. Outside workers involved in counselling or groupwork can have a profound effect on the prisoners they work with and it is important for them to understand the environment in which prisoners live and the pressures of prison life on staff and inmates. *It may be useful for workers to be offered the opportunity to spend a day with prison officers on normal duties before starting work.*

It is often a source of amazement to people in the community working with prisons that different prison departments frequently have little idea what outside contacts their colleagues have. For example, there are prisons where the hospital is totally unaware that drugs agencies have been offering a service (through the probation or pre-release course) for some time. From the outside it often seems that mechanisms for communication about outside agencies and the services they offer are deficient. This may be because of the rather *ad hoc* manner in which such services have evolved in many prisons.

Since more extensive contact with community agencies seems to be an accelerating trend *it may be that one individual in the prison management team should act as a co-ordinating point for external agencies.* The role of this person could be that of contact point and key negotiator responsible for direct liaison with outside bodies. Alternatively, active contact could remain with individual departments with the co-ordinator simply maintaining an updated list of agencies involved and the services provided, so that any new proposals could be considered in the context of work already in progress.

Regular bi-annual or quarterly meetings of representatives from agencies working in the prison with a member of prison staff would also be useful so that any general difficulties could be discussed. There are already 'outsiders' groups involved with some prisons, consisting of people working with the prison. They are often organised independently of the prison, and where they exist they could provide a structure to enable this type of consultation to take place. Another useful role for the co-ordinator might be the production of an information sheet for people wishing to work with the prison. All too often workers have to find out even the most basic facts – such as how to make appointments to see prisoners, whether giving cigarettes to prisoners to smoke during an interview is allowed, and who to contact if an appointment has to be cancelled – by trial and error.

The success or failure of an outside agency's work with a prison often depends on how prisoners gain access to the service. Posters on wing or unit notice boards may be the most obvious means of advertising what is available, but in time they are likely to be defaced or removed. A more dynamic approach, in addition to traditional advertisements and leaflets, may be for all staff with a pastoral role to be fully informed of what is available. This may apply particularly to wing, house or unit staff if they are involved in a personal officer scheme. Perhaps information about services provided by community-based agencies could form part of the training of personal officers. It would also be desirable for them to receive regular updates.

Prisoners wishing to seek help from outside agencies may be deterred if it involves everyone around them being aware that they need advice on drugs, alcohol or HIV. While it is difficult to arrange confidential access within a closed prison, attention should certainly be given to maintaining as much privacy as possible for those wishing to use the service.

Summary

Working with Prisons – a Guide for Community-based Agencies

Preparing for Prison Work

Before embarking on prison work community-based agencies would be well advised to:
– consider why they wish to become involved in prison work;
– decide what service they wish to offer;
– decide how much agency time can be devoted to prison work;
– ensure that a reliable service can be offered;
– consider what impact prison work will have on the other work of the agency;
– determine clear aims for the work, define the boundaries of the agency's commitment and consider the implications for the long-term strategy of the agency.

Making Contact

There is no definitive way of making successful contact with a prison. However it may be useful to:
– use any existing known contact points;
– write a letter to the prison governor outlining what the agency has to offer.

After making initial contact it is advisable to:
– find out what else is happening in the prison with regard to the type of work proposed;
– explore the possibility of spending time with members of various departments in the institution;
– invite any interested prison staff to visit the agency.

Once contact is established and the service to be provided is being negotiated it may help to:

– ensure that all meetings between the prison and the agency are minuted;

– aim at negotiating some form of contract with the prison about the terms on which the service is offered and the expectations of the prison and of the agency;

– consider how prisoners will reach the service and whether this is likely to have any implications for them.

Working with Prisoners

If the agency is offering a service directly to prisoners it is important for workers to bear in mind that:

– many prisoners have little outside contact and an enormous amount of time to think;

– many prisoners spend a lot of time alone. The effect of an upsetting counselling session or group can be compounded by this;

– the boundaries of contact between worker and prisoner need to be established at the outset, reiterated as necessary and adhered to;

– even a small-scale breach of the rules on the worker's part will wreck the chances of that agency continuing to work in the prison and may jeopardise the efforts of other agencies;

– it will be useful for the worker to have an ID card made up;

– it is important that the worker is appropriately dressed;

– promises made to prisoners should be kept and care must be taken not to raise a prisoner's expectations if disappointment is likely;

– it is useful to keep in touch with other agencies involved when acting on behalf of a prisoner;

– if an appointment cannot be kept by the worker it is important to inform the prison and to ask specifically that the prisoner be told;

– it may be as well to phone the prison before setting off to make sure that the visit or session is to go ahead;

– adequate support and supervision of people involved in prison work are of crucial importance.

Working with Community-based Agencies – a Guide for Prisons

Preparing to Work with Outside Agencies

To locate local drug or HIV services contact can be made with:
– national organisations such as the Standing Conference on Drug Abuse or look up HIV-related services in the *National AIDS Manual*;
– Regional or District HIV Prevention Co-ordinators;
– the regional prison broker.

Once contact has been made it may be useful to:
– check the reputation of the agency with other existing contacts in the field or with one of the national organisations;
– negotiate the type of service to be offered and the resource implications for the prison at the outset;
– enable the outside worker to spend a day with prison officers on normal duties before starting work;
– nominate one individual in the prison management team as a co-ordinating point for external agencies.

Conclusion

Although more community-based agencies are now working in prisons than ever before there is still enormous scope for expansion. Long-term successful work demands a high degree of co-operation, trust and respect. It often seems that the power in such a relationship lies with the prison where access can easily be blocked if any difficulty occurs. Prisons should be aware that expert services which improve the regime are being offered to them at no cost and they should treat the service providers accordingly. For their part community-based agencies are sometimes reluctant to consider the extreme difficulty of running a service or working in a prison every day. If the role of outside agencies in prison is to expand, long-term planning must take place instead of working in the rather *ad hoc* and patchy manner which has occurred in the past. This would allow everyone to have a better idea of what is expected and lead to greater trust and co-operation.

Appendices

Appendix 1

Examples of Training Needs Analyses

This section contains two different types of interview guides used both to establish staff training needs and to obtain a picture of the kind of HIV education that has already been carried out in the prison.

Full Interview Schedule

1 What is your job?
2 What are your main duties?
3 Do you have any contact with people who are or might be HIV positive or have AIDS?
4 What do you think are the main ways of passing on HIV?
5 Are there any issues raised by HIV that affect your work? Please give details of what these are and how they affect it (for example, first aid practice, health and safety).
6 Do you feel that you have enough information or knowledge to protect yourself from acquiring HIV?
7 What are your main concerns or worries about HIV or AIDS in your work?
8 Have you had any information or training about HIV or AIDS? Please give details.
9 What did you think of this? How useful was it (for example, did it cover all your informational needs)? Please give details.

Extra Questions for Supervisors or Managers

10 Do you think there is a need for an update on this information? Please give details.
11 As a supervisor/manager, what do you think the main concerns of your staff are in relation to HIV or AIDS?
12 As a supervisor/manager, what do you think are the main skills and knowledge that staff need to have in order to work with HIV or AIDS?

Brief Interview Schedule

1 What is your main job and duties?
2 Do you have any contact with people who are HIV positive or who have AIDS?
3 What is the prison's policy on HIV and AIDS? Give details.
4 Are there any issues/concerns raised by HIV and AIDS that affect your work? For example:
  – health and safety
  – first aid
  – confidentiality
  – support/counselling
  – education
  – induction/pre-release
  – medical care.
5 Have you had any training on HIV and AIDS? Give details of what, when, its usefulness, and whether it has been updated.
6 What work is being carried out in the prison on HIV and AIDS
  – for staff?
  – for prisoners?

Appendix 2

Handout on Training Methods

Jan Mojsa

Groupwork Methods

The purpose of this document is to provide basic ideas to encourage group discussion and exploration of issues. Many training materials use these techniques and they work particularly well in adult learning groups.

You may wish to expand these ideas to fit your own requirements or for more creative groupwork.

The Round Robin

This exercise gives each group member the opportunity to speak without interruption. Each person in the group is asked to make a statement or comment, taking it in turns to give their views. It is helpful to allow individuals time to think about what they want to say and to state that nobody will be forced to say anything if they don't want to.

Example

Round robins are useful at the beginning of a course. You can ask group members to introduce themselves, say where they are from, what they hope to gain from the course and so on. You might use it at the end of a course enabling members to say what they have gained from the course, what they liked and what they disliked.

Round robins can work well after a long debate or discussion – participants can be asked to reflect on what they feel are the major issues that have arisen.

The Pyramid

This method can be used to get everyone in a group involved in a task or discussion. The basic principle is to allow participants to work first individually, then in pairs or fours, eventually feeding back to a group discussion. Participants may feel daunted by group discussions – using the pyramid they can be eased into it or at the very least they will have contributed in the smaller groups.

Example
You wish to focus a discussion on, for example, concerns about HIV infection in the workplace. Ask the group to think about their fears individually, making a note of them if they wish. These are shared with a partner or small group where any common concerns can be noted. Afterwards small group discussions are shared with the whole group.

As facilitator you can encourage the flow of discussion by:

- summarising key points;
- introducing new points;
- clarifying any misunderstandings;
- checking the group is happy with the way the discussion is going.

It is important to check whether certain members are dominating the group to the point of excluding others. General awareness of body language (yawning, fidgeting . . . sleeping!) tells you if the discussion has become exhausted, in which case move on to something new or take a break.

Brainstorm

This exercise can be used to generate lots of ideas on a given topic and is a useful tool for sharing information, particularly in small groups. The topic you wish to brainstorm can be structured as appropriate. Note that the wider the topic the more involved the task of sifting through the generated ideas becomes.

As facilitator you can assist the group to clarify and categorise ideas, bring out issues, highlight problems, view positive aspects and so on.

Example
To increase the chance of all members participating, ask the group to split into smaller groups. Ask them to write, on flipchart paper, all the words they can think of for the sexual parts of the body for example. Bring the group together to share their lists and process as necessary.

Alternatively, ask the group to call out places where young people can find information regarding HIV/AIDS, for example and write the list yourself. Process as you feel appropriate.

Case Study

Case studies enable group members to focus on a particular situation or problem and explore potential solutions. Case studies can be prepared beforehand or suggested by group members drawing on their own experience.

Using these scenarios, participants can individually, or in small groups, think through the implications.

Example

Prepared scenario – a manager at work has told you it is unnecessary to take precautions as detailed in the newly circulated health and safety paper because 'It's a lot of scaremongering.' Ask the group:

- What is your reaction?
- What do you think about it?
- How do you feel?
- What should you or could you do?

A scenario can be given to small groups, ask them to spend a specified amount of time discussing it and share their thoughts with the whole group afterwards.

Role Play

Role plays enable a group to practise a situation which might be of concern, for example, talking to a manager or discussing a sensitive topic. During role plays participants act out a scene and then discuss any feelings or issues that may come from the participants' own experience.

It is important to 'de-role' afterwards. (That means to stop being a character and return to the here and now of the training room.) This can be done by each participant saying who they are, what they like and so on. Thoughts, feelings and issues which emerge can be processed in the group as appropriate.

Carousels

Carousels enable a group to experience diverse reactions and opinions. Hopefully everyone will:

- have an opportunity to answer a number of questions;
- experience their own question being answered in different ways.

To set up a carousel, each participant places their chair so they are facing another participant. The easiest way to do this is to form two lines of chairs facing each other. One line is known as A and the other as B. You may wish to give the group a question you prepared beforehand or ask them to write their own – for example, a question they are unsure of or a situation they find difficult to handle. Line A begins by asking the person opposite their question. You can allow, say, three minutes for B to answer. When the time is up, line B moves along one so each participant is facing a new partner. The question is asked again, and once more the line moves down a place. You can repeat the sequence so that line B has the opportunity to ask their questions.

As facilitator you can process a follow-up discussion – for example, ask the group how they felt, what they noticed and whether they were surprised at anything.

Task Groups

Task groups are particularly helpful when the participants have similar backgrounds. A task group, as the name suggests, is a small group which can focus on a specific task in a given time. Again, the question can be prepared beforehand or generated by participants. It may be helpful to use task groups at the end of a course to encourage:

- action planning;
- problem solving;
- consideration of advantages and disadvantages.

Example
Ask a small group, 'What are the advantages and disadvantages of discussing HIV and AIDS within schools?' Give participants a specified amount of time to discuss the implications and ask them to share their findings with the whole group.

Alternatively, ask a small group to draft a policy proposal to give to their health and safety representative regarding first aid procedure. Again, give the groups a specified amount of time to discuss the implications and ask them to share their findings with the whole group.

Appendix 3

Extracts from the Woolf Report

This appendix consists of two extracts from the Woolf Report (Woolf and Tumim, 1991) that make recommendations about the management of drug abusers and the management of HIV and AIDS.

The Management of Drug Abusers

12.339   In its evidence, the Prison Service noted that between 2,000 and 3,000 inmates each year have been reported by medical officers as having some degree of dependence on drugs at the time of their reception into custody. In 1989, 1,159 drug addicts were notified by prison medical officers in accordance with the Misuse of Drugs Regulations 1973. But the Prison Service noted:

'These figures are recognised as understating the scale of drug usage in respect of people sent to prison.'

12.340   The Prison Service has shown us a draft of Professor Gunn's report on Mentally Disordered Prisoners. The report was commissioned by the Home Office and carried out by the Department of Forensic Psychiatry at the Institute of Psychiatry. It suggests that 'drug dependence is the commonest psychiatric problem in sentenced prisoners'. The report found that the facilities in prisons had failed to keep pace with the scale of the problem.

12.341   Professor Gunn's report points out that, with few exceptions:

'prison doctors regarded drug and alcohol abuse as being outside their area of concern',

and that:

'many prison medical officers lack interest or involvement in the care of substance abusers, whether their primary problem is drugs or alcohol.'

12.342   The research carried out for the purposes of Professor Gunn's report was the most extensive ever conducted. It was however confined to the sentenced prison population only.

12.343   In referring to alcohol dependency/abuse, the report uses as its criterion those for whom 'treatment for a drink problem might be appropriate'. For drug dependency/abuse, the criterion is the 'daily use of drugs of dependency during the six months period prior to the index offence'. The figures do not include cannabis users.

12.344   On this basis, the percentage in Professor Gunn's sample for whom the primary diagnosis was alcohol dependency or abuse among adult males was 8.6%. Among male youths, it was 8.7% and among females it was 4.4%. The respective percentages for a primary diagnosis of drug dependency/abuse were, 10.1% adult males, 6.2% male youths and 24.2% females. Based on his sample findings, Professor Gunn estimates that 20.1% of the adult male sentenced population may be diagnosed as dependent on or abusing substances (drugs, alcohol and, to a much lesser extent, pathological gambling) together with 15.8% of the sentenced male youth population and 28.9% of the sentenced female population.

12.345   The Royal College of Psychiatrists, in its evidence to the Inquiry, pointed out that it was not easy to treat alcoholism or drug dependency. The success rate was low. It would be lower still where there was little desire to co-operate. Nevertheless, the College said:

> 'prison, with its many hours of enforced inactivity and boredom for most inmates, could provide a window of opportunity to help these growing numbers of dependent people – the drug abusers, the alcoholics and the pathological gamblers, who now together constitute a fifth of our sentenced population. Self-help organisations such as Alcoholics Anonymous and Gamblers Anonymous already meet in many prisons. They need encouraging and their work extending – in many prisons there is a waiting list of weeks or months for the "Alcohol Class". Voluntary agencies working with drug addicts and others (such as Lifeline in Manchester) should also be encouraged to contribute their experience, enthusiasm, and links with resources outside the walls'.

12.346   We were helped by evidence from Lifeline. They pointed out that the majority of drug users do not identify themselves on reception for fear of receiving different and unpleasant treatment as a result. In many prisons, drug users were placed in isolation for the period of their withdrawal, during which time they received no medication, or at least no medication which would be considered appropriate by the National Health Service.

Lifeline suggested that:

> 'contact between the Prison Medical Service and their NHS counterparts is rare'.

12.347   Lifeline also drew our attention to the problem of the illicit use of drugs by prisoners, as did NAPO (the National Association of Probation Officers). NAPO told us that a Parliamentary Answer on 20 March 1990 had shown that 617 needles or syringes had been found in prison by staff between 1987 and 1989. But Lifeline suggested that too much reliance should not be put on such statistics. Injecting equipment which was smuggled into prison was widely used, they suggested.

12.348   We are not in a position to confirm or comment on these claims. However, Professor Gunn's report says that, while this may be due to under-reporting, the results of his survey do not suggest that injecting is widespread among former drug users in prison. Most prisoners we spoke to in a number of different prisons and in private discussions suggested to us that so-called 'soft' drugs, such as cannabis, were available to some prisoners. But there was much greater reluctance among prisoners to admit to the presence of the harder drugs referred to by Lifeline.

12.349   The problem of drug abuse had already faced a large number of the prisons we visited in Europe, apparently to a greater extent than in this country.

12.350   We have referred earlier in this section to the units in some prisons in the Netherlands – drug free zones. They provide assistance and an improved regime to prisoners who agree to take part in the programmes and avoid any use of drugs. Lifeline commended this system to us. They suggested that drug free units should also be open to non-abusing inmates to avoid the units turning into Rule 43 ghettos. We propose that the Prison Service should examine the experience in the Netherlands and similar initiatives in Sweden and the United States and, subject to examination, should make provision for drug free units. Such programmes would depend on the Prison Service drawing fully on assistance from outside agencies with experience in dealing with such issues. They would be assisted, as we said earlier, if our recommendation for prisoners' 'contracts' is implemented.

12.351   Professor Gunn in his report makes a number of recommendations in relation to alcohol and drug abuse and dependency. He recommends improving the training of all prison staff. He suggests greater efforts to co-ordinate and improve practice, which at the present time is 'poorly developed, variable and fragmented'. The report suggests that every prison receiving drug users should have available a standard opiate withdrawal regime similar to that found at Holloway Prison. The report considers that there is a need for therapeutic community treatment for both drug abusers and alcohol abusers. In relation to drug abusers, it suggests that this should be based on the Grendon model and that it should only be used for a minority of imprisoned drug users. (Although the report refers to a Grendon model, the report also notes that drug abuse is at present regarded as a 'contra-indication' to acceptance at Grendon itself.)

12.352   Professor Gunn's report also refers to the need for liaison with treatment agencies in the community. It suggests that part of a prisoner's preparation for release should include offering to put the prisoner in touch with such agencies.

12.353   These recommendations in Professor Gunn's report appear to us to be sensible and we commend them. We would specifically endorse a further suggestion by Professor Gunn that there should be an individual (we propose a prison officer) who is responsible for co-ordinating the services provided within a prison establishment and in the locality for drug and alcohol abusers.

The Management of HIV/AIDS

12.354   The Prison Service Medical Directorate provided us with a statement of current Prison Service policy in respect of HIV/AIDS dated March 1990. In summary, this provided that all inmates should be questioned on reception to discover whether they were 'high risk' If it appeared that they were such a risk, they were referred to the medical officer for consultation and possible clinical investigation. Blood tests were available to any inmate who requested it, or where the medical officer advised it and the inmate consented. Inmates taking such a test would be counselled. Inmates who proved positive would be placed under a Viral Infectivity Restriction (VIR).

12.355 The policy statement said that staff with an operational need to know were informed of the presence and identity of inmates who had been placed by the medical officer under VIR. Information about such a categorisation might also be available to the police and others in the criminal justice system.

12.356 In a separate note by the Prison Service Medical Directorate, they told us that under VIR arrangements, medical officers had discretion to place some limitations on the regimes for HIV infected prisoners. They should, for example, be in single accommodation, or in accommodation shared with other identified HIV infected prisoners, albeit on ordinary location. Most, if not all, would be excluded from work in the kitchen or other types of work carrying the risk of blood spillage.

12.357 The Medical Directorate told us that they were concerned that too many infected prisoners were kept in the prison hospital, or in a special wing or unit, instead of on normal location. The decision about the location of such prisoners was left to the discretion of local management.

12.358 The evidence we received expressed deep concern about the Prison Service's treatment of HIV prisoners. It was clear, as the Medical Inspectorate accepted, that many prisons were not meeting the Prison Service's own stated policy. This is:

'To provide as normal a prison life as possible for identified HIV infected prisoners who are well.'

12.359 The Inquiry visited a small, dingy and airless basement unit at Wandsworth Prison which contained a number of inmates who either had HIV or who were awaiting the results of HIV tests. Apart from an hour's exercise, visits to the Library and some classes, they were confined to this small area. They had a television and a small amount of weight-lifting equipment. The only available work was a small amount of mail-bag sewing. The only redeeming feature of the unit was the apparently caring attitude of the prison officers on duty, who did what they could to alleviate the situation.

12.360   It is hardly any wonder that, given the prospect of such conditions, prisoners who may be concerned about the possibility of having the AIDS virus, may be reluctant to express that concern to the prison authorities. We could not imagine conditions more likely to deter a prisoner from doing all in his power to avoid revealing that he was or might be HIV positive than those we saw at Wandsworth. The conditions were a travesty of justice.

12.361   The aim must be to provide decent treatment and opportunities for HIV prisoners. The first way to achieve this must be by ensuring that staff are fully aware of the extent to which HIV presents a risk to themselves or other inmates.

12.362   We were impressed with the approach which we saw at Saughton Prison in Edinburgh. The prison had run an AIDS month during which every member of staff in the prison had received training. Every new recruit received AIDS education. Prison officers were used to train other officers. There were small leaflets available for both staff and inmates. Simple informative posters were in most of the prison wings. The result was that there was not, we understand, the same degree of ostracisation of HIV prisoners as we saw at Wandsworth.

12.363   A local initiative at Bristol Prison has also resulted in a greater awareness by staff of the needs of prisoners with HIV. A network of trained prison officer counsellors has been established. As a result of the programme, we understand that there has been a greater respect for the confidentiality of information about infected prisoners. We would like to see more support and encouragement of initiatives of this kind.

12.364   The Prison Service should give local prison management a clearer remit to meet their responsibilities in the way they deal with AIDS. Area Managers must ensure that the Prison Service's own policy is met. There should be increased efforts to educate prison staff. The examples of good practice we have described might usefully be extended.

12.365   There needs also to be a reassurance for inmates who test positive that they will be given the help and counselling they require. We propose that each prison should ensure that it has the necessary links with AIDS counselling agencies. We envisage such agencies providing skilled assistance to the contribution which prison officers themselves can make to this work.

12.366   The National AIDS Trust, the National AIDS and Prisons Forum and the National Association of Probation Officers recommended that the Viral Infectivity Restriction (VIR) should be abolished as far as it affected the management of HIV positive prisoners. In addition the National AIDS Trust and the AIDS and Prisons Consortium Project recommended that there should be a greater degree of confidentiality than exists at present. This evidence suggested that the identification of a prisoner with HIV/AIDS had no relevance outside the medical field. What was needed instead was proper education on health and safety procedures, and the implementation of those procedures.

12.367   We are clear from the evidence we have seen that the identification of prisoners who are HIV positive by placing them under VIR can result in their being unjustifiably segregated. We have received no evidence to justify these restrictions or to suggest that they are a necessary means of protection in prisons.

12.368   We were told that at Saughton Prison in Edinburgh there was no VIR or equivalent regulation and no formal or informal segregation of prisoners with AIDS and HIV infection. We were impressed too that, when the VIR restriction was withdrawn at Bristol, 24 out of approximately 500 prisoners at Bristol were prepared voluntarily to disclose that they were HIV positive. This compared with Wandsworth, where only 12 of approximately 1,700 prisoners had identified themselves as HIV positive.

12.369   We have no evidence either that disclosure – on a 'need to know' basis – to wing staff that a prisoner was HIV positive is necessary or desirable. We were told that the Prison Services in Europe (most notably France and Switzerland) applied the normal rules of medical confidentiality. At Saughton we were told that neither the Governor nor the prison officers would be given this information. Only the medical staff knew. If the prisoner was transferred, medical information about him was passed through the normal medical channels.

12.370   HIV positive prisoners must not and need not become the pariahs of the prison system. It is in the interests of the prisoner, the prison in which he is serving his sentence and the public that those prisoners who feel they are at risk of being HIV positive identify themselves and co-operate voluntarily with the carrying out of tests.

Prisoners must be able to do so with the knowledge that, if the tests prove positive, they will be helped, not hounded. These must be the central objectives. Unless the Prison Service radically changes its approach there can be no hope of them being met.

12.371   The Prison Service's present policy on confidentiality and VIR is out of accord with the general approach which we have proposed. It could well be counterproductive by encouraging prisoners to conceal the extent to which they are at risk. We are not in a position to form a final view on any medical aspects to the present policies. We note, however, that other jurisdictions appear to do well without them. These are matters on which it is clearly necessary to reassure staff and provide them with clear training and advice. But, ultimately, the Prison Service, on the basis of the best medical advice it can get, must decide the policy. And it must ensure that establishments are not able to [flout] that policy by local practices or agreements.

12.372   We propose that, as soon as possible, there should be a thorough review of the present policies of the Prison Service in relation to HIV. The review should:

(a) subject the present policies in respect of VIR and confidentiality to critical examination with a view to setting them aside;

(b) identify the action which can be taken by establishments to encourage prisoners who feel that they are at risk of being HIV positive to identify themselves and co-operate voluntarily with tests;

(c) draw up a programme of treatment and opportunities for HIV positive prisoners;

(d) examine the best practices which already exist within the Prison Service and the Prison Service in Scotland for training prison officers and then draw up proposals to ensure that the best practices are adopted in all establishments;

(e) consider the best way of achieving close co-operation between prisons and AIDS counselling agencies.

12.373   When the review has been completed, a new policy on HIV should be announced by the Prison Service. The importance of implementing that policy should be forcefully drawn to the attention of Area Managers and Governors.

Appendix 4

Useful Training Resources

Aggleton P., Homans H., Mojsa J., Watson S. and Watney S. *Learning About AIDS* (Churchill Livingstone, Edinburgh, 1988). Exercises and materials for adult education about HIV/AIDS.

Aggleton P., Horsley C., Warwick I. and Wilton T. *AIDS Working With Young People* (AIDS Education and Research Trust, Horsham, 1990).

AIDS Inside and Out (Home Office, London, 1989). A manual for tutors which accompanies the Prison Department video.

Bain P., Gale W., and Taylor R. *HIV and AIDS: a Training Pack for Young People: 16–19 Years* (Liverpool Health Authority, Liverpool, 1989).

Cranfield S. and Dixon A. *Drug Training, HIV and AIDS in the 1990s* (Health Education Authority, London, 1990).

Dixon H. and Gordon P. *Working With Uncertainty* (Family Planning Education Unit, London, 1988).

Lockley P. and Williams M. *HIV/AIDS Counselling: Trainer's Pack* (Scottish Health Education Group, Edinburgh – now Health Education Board for Scotland, 1989).

Appendix 5

Part 1: Directory of Prisons and Young Offender Institutions (YOIs), with corresponding District Health Authorities

The left-hand column lists prisons and YOIs alphabetically. The right-hand column lists the health districts in which they are located.

The *contact* telephone number should put you in touch with the person or department responsible for HIV/AIDS health education within the district. They might be referred to as 'HIV Prevention Co-ordinators', 'AIDS Liaison Officers' or 'Health Promotion Officers'.

*** Indicates a women's prison or YOI.*

Prison or YOI	District Health Authority HQ
Acklington Morpeth Northumberland NE65 9XF Tel: (0670) 760411	**Northumberland** East Cottingwood Morpeth Northumberland NE61 2PD Tel: (0670) 514331 Contact Tel: (0670) 514331
Albany Newport Isle of Wight PO30 5RS Tel: (0983) 524055	**Isle of Wight** Whitecroft Hospital Sandy Lane Newport Isle of Wight PO30 3ED Tel: (0983) 526011 Contact Tel: (0983) 524233
Aldington Ashford Kent TN25 7BQ Tel: (023) 372436/7 & 372796	**South East Kent** Ash-Eton Radnor Park West Folkestone Kent CT19 5HL Tel: (0303) 850202 Contact Tel: (0303) 851127

Ashwell
Oakham
Leicestershire LE15 7LS
Tel: (0572) 756075

Askham Grange**
Askham Richard
York YO2 3PT
Tel: (0904) 704236–8

Aylesbury (YOI)
Bierton Road
Aylesbury
Buckinghamshire HP20 1EH
Tel: (0296) 24435

Bedford
St Loyes Street
Bedford MK40 1HG
Tel: (0234) 358671

Belmarsh
Western Way
Thamesmead
Woolwich
London SE28 0EB
Tel: (081) 317 2436

Birmingham
Winson Green Road
Birmingham B18 4AS
Tel: (021) 554 3838

Blantyre House
Gouldhurst
Cranbrook
Kent TN17 2NA
Tel: (0580) 211367

Blundeston
Lowestoft
Suffolk NR32 5BG
Tel: (0502) 730591

Leicestershire
20/28 Princess Road West
Leicester LE1 6TY
Tel: (0533) 559777
Contact Tel: (0533) 559777 x 8541

York
Bootham Park
York YO3 7BY
Tel: (0904) 610700
Contact Tel: (0904) 637490

Aylesbury Vale
Ardenham Lane
Aylesbury
Buckinghamshire HP19 3DX
Tel: (0296) 437501
Contact Tel: (0296) 437571

North Bedfordshire
3 Kimbolton Road
Bedford MK40 2NU
Tel: (0234) 355122
Contact Tel: (0234) 355122 x 3465

Greenwich
Memorial Hospital
Shooters Hill
London SE18 3RZ
Tel: (081) 856 5511
Contact Tel: (081) 858 8141 x 2143

West Birmingham
Dudley Road Hospital
Dudley Road
Birmingham B18 7QH
Tel: (021) 554 3801
Contact Tel: (021) 554 3899 x 243

Tunbridge Wells
Sherwood Park
Pembury Road
Tunbridge Wells
Kent TN2 3QE
Tel: (0892) 511577
Contact Tel: (0892) 39144 x 49

Great Yarmouth & Waveney
Northgate Hospital
Northgate Street
Great Yarmouth
Norfolk NR30 1BU
Tel: (0493) 850411
Contact Tel: (0493) 856222 x 350

Brinsford (YOI)
New Road
Featherstone
Wolverhampton WV10 7PU
Tel: (0902) 791118

Mid-Staffordshire
Mellor House
Corporation Street
Stafford
Staffordshire ST16 3SR
Tel: (0785) 222888
Contact Tel: (0785) 222888 x 5246

Bristol
Cambridge Road
Bristol BS7 8PS
Tel: (0272) 426661

Bristol
Manulife House
2 Marlborough Street
Bristol BS1 3NP
Tel: (0272) 290666
Contact Tel: (0272) 290666 x 206

Brixton
PO Box 369
Jebb Avenue
Brixton
London SW2 5XF
Tel: (081) 674 9811

West Lambeth
St Thomas' Hospital
Lambeth Palace Road
London SE1 7EH
Tel: (071) 928 9292
Contact Tel: (071) 955 4386

Brockhill
Redditch
Worcestershire B97 6RD
Tel: (0527) 550314

Bromsgrove/Redditch
165a Birmingham Road
Worcestershire B61 0DJ
Tel: (0527) 73285
Contact Tel: (0527) 36903

Bullingdon
Patrick Haugh Road
Arncott
Bicester
Oxon OX6 0PZ
Tel: (0869) 321367/8

Oxfordshire
Manor House
Headley Way
Headington
Oxford OX3 9DZ
Tel: (0865) 741741
Contact Tel: (0865) 222138

Bullwood Hall (YOI and Prison)**
High Road
Hockley
Essex SS5 4TE
Tel: (0702) 202515

Southend
Union Lane
Rochford
Essex SS4 1RB
Tel: (0702) 546354
Contact Tel: (0702) 546354 x 381

Camp Hill
Newport
Isle of Wight
PO30 5PB
Tel: (0983) 527661

Isle of Wight
Whitecroft Hospital
Sandy Lane
Newport
Isle of Wight PO30 3ED
Tel: (0983) 526011
Contact Tel: (0983) 524233

Canterbury
Longport
Canterbury
Kent CT1 1PJ
Tel: (0227) 762244

Canterbury & Thanet
Regency Buildings
3 Royal Crescent
Ramsgate
Kent CT11 9PF
Tel: (0843) 594592
Contact Tel: (0843) 594592 x 5305

Cardiff
Knox Road
Cardiff
Glamorgan CF2 1UG
Tel: (0222) 491212

Castington
Morpeth
Northumberland NE65 9XG
Tel: (0670) 760942

Channings Wood
Denbury
Newton Abbot
Devon TQ12 6DW
Tel: (0803) 812361

Chelmsford
Springfield Road
Chelmsford
Essex CM2 6LQ
Tel: (0245) 268651

Coldingley
Bisley
Woking
Surrey GU24 9EX
Tel: (04867) 6721

Cookham Wood**
Rochester
Kent ME1 3LU
Tel: (0634) 814981

Dartmoor
Princetown
Yelverton
Devon PL20 6RR
Tel: (082 289) 261

Deerbolt (YOI)
Bowes Road
Barnard Castle
Co Durham DL12 9BG
Tel: (0833) 37561

South Glamorgan
Temple of Peace and Health
Cathays Park
Cardiff CF1 3NW
Tel: (0222) 231021
Contact Tel: (0222) 522011

Northumberland
East Cottingwood
Morpeth
Northumberland NE61 2PD
Tel: (0670) 514331
Contact Tel: (0670) 514331

Exeter
Dean Clarke House
Southernhay East
Exeter EX1 1PR
Tel: (0392) 411222
Contact Tel: (0392) 406106

Mid Essex
Collingwood Road
Witham
Essex CM8 2TT
Tel: (0376) 516515
Contact Tel: (0245) 490089

West Surrey & NE Hants
3rd Floor Abbey House
283–92 Farnborough Road
Farnborough
Hampshire GU14 7NE
Tel: (0252) 548881
Contact Tel: (0276) 692211 x 6260

Medway
District HQ
Medway Hospital
Windmill Road
Gillingham
Kent ME7 5NY
Tel: (0634) 830000
Contact Tel: (0634) 830000 x 3532

Plymouth
Derriford Business Park
Brest Road
Derriford
Plymouth PL6 5XN
Tel: (0752) 793793
Contact Tel: (0752) 367131

Darlington
Memorial Hospital
Hollyhurst Road
Darlington DL3 6HX
Tel: (0325) 380100
Contact Tel: (0325) 380100 x 3082

Dorchester
North Square
Dorchester
Dorset DT1 1JD
Tel: (0305) 266021

West Dorset
Somerleigh Gate
Dorset County Hospital
Princes Street
Dorchester DT1 1TS
Tel: (0305) 263123
Contact Tel: (0305) 779224

Dover (YOI)
The Citadel
Western Heights
Dover
Kent CT17 9DR
Tel: (0304) 203848

South East Kent
Ash-Eton
Radnor Park West
Folkestone
Kent CT19 5HL
Tel: (0303) 850202
Contact Tel: (0303) 851127

Downview
Sutton Lane
Sutton
Surrey SM2 5PD
Tel: (081) 770 7500

Merton & Sutton
6 Homeland Drive
Sutton
Surrey SM2 5LY
Tel: (081) 685 9922
Contact Tel: (081) 685 9922 x 3294

Drake Hall (YOI and Prison)**
Eccleshall
Staffs ST21 6LQ
Tel: (0785) 850621

North Staffordshire
North Staffordshire Royal Infirmary
Princes Road
Hartshill
Stoke on Trent ST4 7JN
Tel: (0782) 49144
Contact Tel: (0782) 716711

Durham (contains one wing for women)
Old Elvet
Durham DH1 3HU
Tel: (091) 386 2621

Durham
District HQ
Appleton House
Lanchester Road
Durham DH1 5XZ
Tel: (091) 386 4911
Contact Tel: (091) 386 4911 x 3365

East Sutton Park (YOI and Prison)**
Sutton Valence
Maidstone
Kent ME17 3DF
Tel: (0622) 842711

Maidstone
Preston Hall
Maidstone
Kent ME20 7NJ
Tel: (0622) 710161
Contact Tel: (0622) 710161 x 3024

Eastwood Park (YOI)
Church Avenue
Falfield
Wotton-under-Edge
Gloucestershire GL12 8DB
Tel: (0454) 260771

Southmead
Southmead General Hospital
Westbury-on-Trym
Bristol BS10 5NB
Tel: (0272) 505050
Contact Tel: (0272) 290666 x 206

Erlestoke House
Devizes
Wiltshire SN10 5TU
Tel: (0380) 813475

Bath & District
Newbridge Hill
Bath
Avon BA1 3QE
Tel: (0225) 313640
Contact Tel: (0225) 313640 x 330

Everthorpe (YOI)
Brough
North Humberside HU15 1RB
Tel: (0430) 422471

Exeter
New North Road
Exeter
Devon EX4 4EX
Tel: (0392) 78321

Featherstone
New Road
Featherstone
Wolverhampton WV10 7PU
Tel: (0902) 790991

Feltham (YOI)
Bedfont Road
Feltham
Middlesex TW13 4ND
Tel: (081) 890 0061

Finnamore Wood (YOI)
Frieth Road
Medmenham
Marlow
Buckinghamshire SL7 2HX
Tel: (0494) 881275

Ford
Arundel
West Sussex BN18 0BX
Tel: (0903) 717261

Foston Hall
Foston
Derbyshire DE6 5DN
Tel: (0283) 585511

East Yorkshire
West House
Westwood Hospital
Beverley HU17 8BU
Tel: (0482) 875875
Contact Tel: (0482) 875875

Exeter
Dean Clarke House
Southernhay East
Exeter EX1 1PR
Tel: (0392) 411222
Contact Tel: (0392) 406106

Mid Staffordshire
Mellor House
Corporation Street
Stafford ST16 3SR
Tel: (0785) 222888
Contact Tel: (0785) 222888 x 5246

Hounslow & Spelthorne
92 Bath Road
Hounslow
Middlesex TW3 3EL
Tel: (081) 570 7715
Contact Tel: (081) 570 7715 x 2243

Wycombe
Oakengrove
Shrubbery Road
High Wycombe
Buckinghamshire HP13 6PS
Tel: (0494) 526161
Contact Tel: (0494) 473888

Chichester
PO Box 42
Royal West Sussex Hospital
Broyle Road
Chichester
West Sussex PO19 4AS
Tel: (0243) 781411
Contact Tel: (0243) 781411 x 235

Southern Derbyshire
Boden House
Main Centre
Derbyshire DE1 2PH
Tel: (0332) 363971
Contact Tel: (0332) 44134

Frankland
PO Box 40
Frankland
Low Newton
Brasside
Durham DH1 5YF
Tel: (091) 384 5544

Full Sutton
Moor Lane
Full Sutton
Nr Stamford Bridge
York YO4 1PS
Tel: (0759) 72447

Garth
Ulnes Walton Lane
Preston
Lancashire PR5 3NE
Tel: (0772) 622722

Gartree
Leicester Road
Market Harborough
Leicester LE16 7RP
Tel: (0858) 410234

Glen Parva (YOI)
Tigers Road
Wigston
Leicestershire LE8 2TN
Tel: (0533) 772022

Gloucester
Barrack Square
Gloucester GL1 2JN
Tel: (0452) 529551

Grendon
Grendon Underwood
Aylesbury
Buckinghamshire HP18 0TL
Tel: (0296) 770301

Guys Marsh (YOI)
Shaftesbury
Dorset SP7 0AH
Tel: (0747) 53344

Durham
District HQ
Appleton House
Lanchester Road
Durham DH1 5XZ
Tel: (091) 386 4911
Contact Tel: (091) 386 4911 x 3365

East Yorkshire
West House
Westwood Hospital
Beverley HU17 8BU
Tel: (0482) 875875
Contact Tel: (0482) 875875

Chorley & South Ribble
District Offices
Chorley & District General Hospital
Preston Road
Chorley PR7 1PP
Tel: (0257) 261222
Contact Tel: (0257) 245325

Leicestershire
20/28 Princess Road West
Leicester LE1 6TY
Tel: (0533) 559777
Contact Tel: (0533) 559777 x 8541

Leicestershire
20/28 Princess Road West
Leicester LE1 6TY
Tel: (0533) 559777
Contact Tel: (0533) 559777 x 8541

Gloucester
Rikenel
Montpellier
Gloucester GL1 1LY
Tel: (0452) 294211
Contact Tel: (0242) 222222

Aylesbury Vale
Ardenham Lane
Aylesbury
Buckinghamshire HP19 3DX
Tel: (0296) 437501
Contact Tel: (0296) 437501 x 258

West Dorset
Somerleigh Gate
Dorset County Hospital
Prince's Street
Dorchester DT1 1TS
Tel: (0305) 263123
Contact Tel: (0305) 779224

Haslar (YOI)
Gosport
Hampshire PO12 2AW
Tel: (0705) 580381

Hatfield (YOI)
Doncaster
South Yorkshire DN7 6EL
Tel: (0405) 812336

Haverigg
Haverigg Camp
Millom
Cumbria LA18 4NA
Tel: (0229) 772131

Hewell Grange (YOI)
Redditch
Worcestershire B97 6QQ
Tel: (0527) 550843

Highpoint
Stradishall
Newmarket
Suffolk CB8 9YG
Tel: (0440) 820611

Hindley
Gibson Street
Bickershaw
Hindley
Wigan
Lancashire WN2 5TH
Tel: (0942) 866255

Hollesley Bay (YOI)
Hollesley Bay Colony
Woodbridge
Suffolk IP12 3JS
Tel: (0394) 411741

Holloway**
Parkhurst Road
Holloway
London N7 0NU
Tel: (071) 607 6747

Portsmouth & SE Hampshire
St Mary's Hospital
Milton Road
Portsmouth PO3 6AD
Tel: (0705) 822331
Contact Tel: (0705) 480144

Doncaster
York House
Cleveland Street
Doncaster DN1 3EJ
Tel: (0302) 367051
Contact Tel: (0302) 854661 x 35

South Cumbria
Priors Lea
Abbey Road
Barrow-in-Furness
Tel: (0229) 870870
Contact Tel: (0229) 870870

Bromsgrove/Redditch
165a Birmingham Road
Bromsgrove
Worcestershire B61 0DJ
Tel: (0527) 73285
Contact Tel: (0527) 36903

West Suffolk
Thingoe House
Cotton Lane
Bury St Edmunds
Suffolk IP33 1YJ
Tel: (0284) 702544
Contact Tel: (0284) 763131

Wigan
Bryan House
61 Standishgate
Wigan WN1 1UP
Tel: (0942) 44000
Contact Tel: (0942) 822763

East Suffolk
PO Box 55
St Clement's Hospital
Foxhall Road
Ipswich IP3 8NN
Tel: (0473) 712272
Contact Tel: (0473) 720931 x 240

Islington
Dartmouth Park Hill
London N19 5HT
Tel: (071) 272 3070
Contact Tel: (071) 387 1908

Hull
Hedon Road
Hull
North Humberside HU9 5LS
Tel: (0482) 20673

Huntercombe (YOI)
Huntercombe Place
Nuffield
Henley-on-Thames
Oxon RG9 5SB
Tel: (0491) 641711

Kingston
Milton Road
Portsmouth
Hampshire PO3 6AS
Tel: (0705) 829561

Kirkham
Preston
Lancashire PR4 2RA
Tel: (0772) 684343

Kirklevington Grange (YOI)
Yarm
Cleveland TS15 9PA
Tel: (0642) 781391

Lancaster
The Castle
Lancaster LA1 1YL
Tel: (0524) 68871

Latchmere House
Church Road
Ham Common
Richmond
Surrey TW10 5HH
Tel: (081) 948 0215

Leeds
Armley
Leeds
West Yorkshire LS12 2TJ
Tel: (0532) 636411

Hull
Victoria House
Park Street
Hull HU2 8TD
Tel: (0482) 223191
Contact Tel: (0482) 875875 x 3128

West Berkshire
Prospect Park Hospital
Honey End Lane
Tilehurst
Reading RG3 4EJ
Tel: (0734) 586161
Contact Tel: (0734) 586161

Portsmouth & SE Hampshire
St Mary's Hospital
Milton Road
Portsmouth PO3 6AD
Tel: (0705) 822331
Contact Tel: (0705) 480144

Preston
District HQ
Watling Street
Fulwood
Preston PR2 4DX
Tel: (0772) 716565
Contact Tel: (0772) 711215

North Tees
North Tees General Hospital
Hardwick
Stockton-on-Tees TS19 8PE
Tel: (0642) 672122
Contact Tel: (0642) 677701

Lancaster
Lancaster Moor Hospital
Lancaster LA1 3JR
Tel: (0524) 65241
Contact Tel: (0524) 35933

Richmond, Twickenham & Roehampton
Queen Mary's University Hospital
Roehampton SW15 5PN
Tel: (081) 789 6611
Contact Tel: (081) 943 4177

Leeds Western
Leeds General Infirmary
Great George Street
Leeds LS1 3EX
Tel: (0532) 432799
Contact Tel: (0532) 781341 x 443

Leicester
Welford Road
Leicester LE2 7AJ
Tel: (0533) 546911

Lewes
Brighton Road
Lewes
East Sussex BN7 1EA
Tel: (0273) 477331

Leyhill
Wotton-under-Edge
Gloucestershire GL12 8HL
Tel: (0454) 260681

Lincoln
Greetwell Road
Lincoln LN2 4BD
Tel: (0522) 533633

Lindholme
Bawtry Road
Hatfield Woodhouse
Doncaster DN7 6EE
Tel: (0302) 846600

Littlehey
Perry
Huntingdon
Cambridge PE18 0SR
Tel: (0480) 812202

Liverpool
68 Hornby Road
Liverpool L9 3DF
Tel: (051) 525 5971

Long Lartin
South Littleton
Evesham
Worcestershire WR11 5TZ
Tel: (0386) 830101

Leicestershire
20/28 Princess Road West
Leicester LE1 6TY
Tel: (0533) 559777
Contact Tel: (0533) 559777 x 8541

Brighton
Brighton General Hospital
Elm Grove
Brighton
Sussex BN2 3EW
Tel: (0273) 696011
Contact Tel: (0273) 696011 x 3775

Southmead
Southmead General Hospital
Westbury-on-Trym
Bristol BS10 5NB
Tel: (0272) 505050
Contact Tel: (0272) 290666 x 206

North Lincolnshire
Cross O'Cliff Court
Bracebridge Heath
Lincoln LN4 2HL
Tel: (0522) 532321
Contact Tel: (0522) 532321 x 204

Doncaster
York House
Cleveland Street
Doncaster DN1 3EJ
Tel: (0302) 367051
Contact Tel: (0302) 854661 x 35

Huntingdon
Primrose Lane
Huntingdon
Cambridgeshire PE18 6SE
Tel: (0480) 450571
Contact Tel: (0480) 457131 x 231

South Sefton
District HQ
Fazackerley Hospital
Longmoor Lane
Liverpool L9 7AL
Tel: (051) 525 3622
Contact Tel: (051) 733 4020 x 2507

Worcester & District
Isaac Maddox House
Shrub Hill Road
Worcester WR4 9RW
Tel: (0905) 763333
Contact Tel: (0905) 229557

Low Newton**
Brasside
Durham DH1 5SD
Tel: (091) 386 1141

Durham
District HQ
Appleton House
Lanchester Road
Durham DH1 5XZ
Tel: (091) 386 4911
Contact Tel: (091) 386 4911 x 3365

Maidstone
County Road
Maidstone
Kent ME14 1UZ
Tel: (0622) 755611

Preston Hall
Maidstone
Kent ME20 7NJ
Tel: (0622) 710161
Contact Tel: (0622) 710161 x 3024

Manchester
Southall Street
Manchester M60 9AH
Tel: (061) 834 8626

North Manchester
North Manchester General Hospital
Crumpsall
Manchester M8 6RL
Tel: (061) 795 4567
Contact Tel: (061) 205 2393 x 216

Moorland (YOI)
Bawtry Road
Hatfield Woodhouse
Doncaster
South Yorkshire DN7 6BW
Tel: (0302) 351500

Doncaster
York House
Cleveland Street
Doncaster DN1 3EJ
Tel: (0302) 367051
Contact Tel: (0302) 854661 x 35

Morton Hall
Swinderby
Lincoln LN6 9PS
Tel: (0522) 868151

North Lincolnshire
Cross O'Cliff Court
Bracebridge Heath
Lincoln LN4 2HL
Tel: (0522) 532321
Contact Tel: (0522) 532321 x 204

The Mount
Molyneaux Avenue
Bovingdon
Herts HP3 0NZ
Tel: (0442) 834363

North West Hertfordshire
99 Waverley Road
St Albans
Hertfordshire AL3 5TL
Tel: (0727) 866122
Contact Tel: (0727) 866122 x 4801

New Hall (YOI and Prison)**
Dial Wood
Flockton
Wakefield
West Yorkshire WF4 4AX
Tel: (0924) 848307

Wakefield
District HQ
Stanley Royd Hospital
Aberford Road
Wakefield WF1 4DH
Tel: (0924) 375217
Contact Tel: (0924) 375217 x 2251

Northallerton (YOI)
East Road
Northallerton
North Yorkshire DL6 1NW
Tel: (0609) 780078

Northallerton
District HQ
Friarage Hospital
Northallerton DL6 1JG
Tel: (0609) 779911
Contact Tel: (0609) 779911 x 712514

Northeye
Barnhorn Road
Bexhill-on-Sea
East Sussex TN39 4QW
Tel: (04243) 5511

North Sea Camp
Freiston
Boston
Lincolnshire PE22 0QX
Tel: (0205) 760481

Norwich
Mousehold
Norwich
Norfolk NR1 4LU
Tel: (0603) 37531

Nottingham
Perry Road
Sherwood
Nottingham NG5 3AG
Tel: (0602) 625022

Onley (YOI)
Willoughby
Rugby
Warwickshire CV23 8AP
Tel: (0788) 522022

Oxford
New Road
Oxford OX1 1LX
Tel: (0865) 721261

Parkhurst
Newport
Isle of Wight PO30 5NX
Tel: (0983) 523855

Pentonville
Caledonian Road
London N7 8TT
Tel: (071) 607 5353

Hastings
St Anne's House
729 The Ridge
St Leonards-on-Sea
Sussex TN37 7PT
Tel: (0424) 754488
Contact Tel: (0424) 720444 x 223

South Lincolnshire
Eastgate
Sleaford
Lincolnshire NG34 7EB
Tel: (0529) 414166
Contact Tel: (0529) 8685

Norwich
St Andrews Hospital (North Side)
Yarmouth Road
Norwich NR7 0SS
Tel: (0603) 300600
Contact Tel: (0603) 613435

Nottingham
Forest House
Berkeley Avenue
Nottingham NG3 5AF
Tel: (0602) 691691
Contact Tel: (0602) 691691 x 49315

Rugby
24 Warwick Street
Rugby CV21 3DH
Tel: (0788) 572831
Contact Tel: (0788) 572831 x 4228

Oxfordshire
Manor House
Headley Way
Headington
Oxford OX3 9DZ
Tel: (0865) 741741
Contact Tel: (0865) 222138

Isle of Wight
Whitecroft Hospital
Sandy Lane
Newport
Isle of Wight PO30 3ED
Tel: (0983) 526011
Contact Tel: (0983) 524233

Islington
Dartmouth Park Hill
London N19 5HT
Tel: (071) 272 3070
Contact Tel: (071) 387 1908

Portland (YOI)
Easton
Portland
Dorset DT5 1DL
Tel: (0305) 820301

Prescoed (YOI)
Coed-y-Paen
Pontypool
NP4 0TD
Tel: (02913) 2231

Preston
2 Ribbleton Lane
Preston
Lancashire PR1 5AB
Tel: (0772) 57734

Pucklechurch**
Bristol BS17 3QJ
Tel: (027582) 2606

Ranby
Retford
Nottinghamshire DN22 8EU
Tel: (0777) 706721

Reading
Forbury Road
Reading
Berkshire RG1 3HY
Tel: (0734) 587031

Risley**
Warrington Road
Risley
Warrington
Cheshire WA3 6BP
Tel: (0925) 763871

West Dorset
Somerleigh Gate
Dorset County Hospital
Prince's Street
Dorchester DT1 1TS
Tel: (0305) 263123
Contact Tel: (0305) 779224

Gwent
Mamhilad
Pontypool
Gwent NP4 0YP
Tel: (0495) 762401
Contact Tel: (0633) 430300

Preston
District HQ
Watling Street
Fulwood
Preston PR2 4DX
Tel: (0772) 716565
Contact Tel: (0772) 711215

Frenchay
Beckspool Road
Frenchay Common
Bristol BS16 1ND
Tel: (0272) 701070
Contact Tel: (0272) 701070

Bassetlaw
Blythe Road
Worksop
Nottinghamshire S81 0BD
Tel: (0777) 705261
Contact Tel: (0777) 705261

West Berkshire
Prospect Park Hospital
Honey End Lane
Tilehurst
Reading RG3 4EJ
Tel: (0734) 586161
Contact Tel: (0734) 586161 x 2318

Warrington
District HQ
Winwick Hospital
Winwick
Warrington
Cheshire WA2 8RR
Tel: (0925) 36151
Contact Tel: (0925) 51188 x 3844

Rochester (YOI)
Rochester
Kent ME1 3QS
Tel: (0634) 830300

Rudgate
Wetherby
West Yorkshire LS23 7AZ
Tel: (0937) 844844

Send
Ripley Road
Woking
Surrey GU23 7LJ
Tel: (0483) 223048

Shepton Mallet
Cornhill
Shepton Mallet
Somerset BA4 5LU
Tel: (0749) 343377

Shrewsbury
The Dana
Shrewsbury
Salop SY1 2HR
Tel: (0743) 352511

Spring Hill
Grendon Underwood
Aylesbury HP18 0TH
Tel: (0296) 770301

Stafford
54 Gaol Road
Stafford ST16 3AW
Tel: (0785) 54421

Medway
District HQ
Medway Hospital
Windmill Road
Gillingham
Kent ME7 5NY
Tel: (0634) 830000
Contact Tel: (0634) 830000 x 3531

Harrogate
Ebor Rise
Cornwall Road
Harrogate HG1 2PU
Tel: (0423) 506141
Contact Tel: (0423) 506141

South West Surrey
Farnham Road Hospital
Guildford
Surrey
Tel: (0483) 61612
Contact Tel: (0483) 37007

Somerset
Wellsprings Road
Taunton
Somerset TA2 7PQ
Tel: (0823) 333491
Contact Tel: (0823) 333491 x 4249

Shropshire
Cross Houses Hospital
Cross Houses
Shrewsbury
Shropshire SY5 6JN
Tel: (0743) 352277
Contact Tel: (0743) 761242 x 509

Aylesbury Vale
Ardenham Lane
Aylesbury
Buckinghamshire HP19 3DX
Tel: (0296) 437501
Contact Tel: (0296) 437501 x 258

Mid-Staffordshire
Mellor House
Corporation Street
Stafford ST16 3SR
Tel: (0785) 222888
Contact Tel: (0785) 222888 x 5246

Standford Hill
Church Road
Eastchurch
Sheerness
Kent ME12 4AA
Tel: (0795) 880441

Stocken
Stocken Hall Road
Stretton
Nr Oakham
Leicestershire LE15 7RD
Tel: (0780) 410771

Stoke Heath (YOI)
Market Drayton
Salop TF9 2JL
Tel: (0630) 654231

Styal (YOI and Prison)**
Wilmslow
Cheshire SK9 4HR
Tel: (0625) 532141

Sudbury
Derbyshire DE6 5HW
Tel: (0283) 585511

Swaleside
Brabazon Road
Eastchurch
Sheerness
Kent ME12 4DZ
Tel: (0795) 880766

Swansea
Oystermouth Road
Swansea
Glamorgan SA1 2SR
Tel: (0792) 464030

Medway
District HQ
Medway Hospital
Windmill Street
Gillingham
Kent ME7 5NY
Tel: (0634) 830000
Contact Tel: (0634) 830000 x 3531

Leicestershire
20/28 Princess Road West
Leicester LE1 6TY
Tel: (0533) 559777
Contact Tel: (0533) 559777 x 8541

Shropshire
Cross Houses Hospital
Cross Houses
Shrewsbury
Shropshire SY5 6JN
Tel: (0743) 352277
Contact Tel: (0743) 761242 x 509

Macclesfield
Macclesfield Hospital
West Park Branch
Prestbury Road
Macclesfield
Cheshire SK10 3BL
Tel: (0625) 210000
Contact Tel: (0625) 661869

Southern Derbyshire
Boden House
Main Centre
Derby DE1 2PH
Tel: (0332) 363971
Contact Tel: (0332) 44134

Medway
District HQ
Medway Hospital
Windmill Road
Gillingham
Kent ME7 5NY
Tel: (0634) 830000
Contact Tel: (0634) 830000 x 3531

West Glamorgan
36 Orchard Street
Swansea SA1 5AQ
Tel: (0792) 458066
Contact Tel: (0792) 471282

Swinfen Hall (YOI)
Lichfield
Staffordshire WS14 9QS
Tel: (0543) 481229

Thorn Cross (YOI)
Arley Road
Appleton
Warrington WA4 4RL
Tel: (0925) 602081

Thorp Arch
Wetherby
West Yorkshire LS23 7AY
Tel: (0937) 844241

Usk
47 Maryport Street
Usk
Gwent NP5 1XP
Tel: (02913) 2411

The Verne
Portland
Dorset DT5 1EQ
Tel: (0305) 820124

Wakefield
Love Lane
Wakefield
West Yorkshire WF2 9AG
Tel: (0924) 378282

Wandsworth
PO Box 757
Heathfield Road
Wandsworth
London SW18 3HS
Tel: (081) 874 7292

South East Staffordshire
Robert Bewick House
Burton District Hospital Centre
Belvedere Road
Burton-on-Trent
Tel: (0283) 66333
Contact Tel: (021) 456 1444

Warrington
District HQ
Winwick Hospital
Winwick
Warrington
Cheshire WA2 8RR
Tel: (0925) 36151
Contact Tel: (0925) 51188 x 3844

Harrogate
Ebor Rise
Cornwall Road
Harrogate HG1 2PU
Tel: (0423) 506141
Contact Tel: (0423) 506141

Gwent
Mamhilad
Pontypool
Gwent NP4 0YP
Tel: (0495) 762401
Contact Tel: (0633) 430300

West Dorset
Somerleigh Gate
Dorset County Hospital
Prince's Street
Dorchester DT1 1TS
Tel: (0305) 263123
Contact Tel: (0305) 779224

Wakefield
District HQ
Stanley Royd Hospital
Aberford Road
Wakefield WF1 4DH
Tel: (0924) 375217
Contact Tel: (0924) 375217 x 2251

Wandsworth
Grosvenor Wing
St George's Hospital
Blackshaw Road
London SW17 0QT
Tel: (081) 672 1255
Contact Tel: (081) 672 6238

Wayland
Griston
Thetford
Norfolk IP25 6RL
Tel: (0953) 884103

Wellingborough
Millers Park
Doddington Road
Wellingborough
Northamptonshire NN8 2NH
Tel: (0933) 224151

Werrington (YOI)
Werrington House
Werrington
Stoke-on-Trent
Staffordshire ST9 0DX
Tel: (078130) 3514

Wetherby (YOI)
York Road
Wetherby
West Yorkshire LS22 5ED
Tel: (0937) 585141

Whatton
Nottingham NG13 9FQ
Tel: (0949) 50511

Whitemore
Longhill Road
March
Nr Peterborough
Cambridgeshire
Tel: (0354) 660653

Winchester
Romsey Road
Winchester
Hampshire SO22 5DF
Tel: (0962) 854494

Wormwood Scrubs
PO Box 757
Du Cane Road
London W12 0AE
Tel: (081) 743 0311

Norwich
St Andrew's Hospital (North Side)
Yarmouth Road
Norwich NR7 0SS
Tel: (0603) 300600
Contact Tel: (0603) 613435

Kettering
The General Hospital
Rothwell Road
Kettering
Northamptonshire NN16 8UZ
Tel: (0536) 523743
Contact Tel: (0536) 492000 x 2565

North Staffordshire
North Staffordshire Royal Infirmary
Princes Road
Hartshill
Stoke-on-Trent ST4 7JN
Tel: (0782) 49144
Contact Tel: (0782) 716711

Harrogate
Ebor Rise
Cornwall Road
Harrogate HG1 2PU
Tel: (0423) 506141
Contact Tel: (0423) 506141

Nottingham
Forest House
Berkeley Avenue
Nottingham NG3 5AF
Tel: (0602) 691691
Contact Tel: (0602) 691691 x 49315

Peterborough
41 Priestgate
Peterborough PE1 1LN
Tel: (0733) 51461
Contact Tel: (0733) 312931 x 163

Winchester
King's Walk
Silver Hill
Winchester SO23 8AF
Tel: (0962) 68111
Contact Tel: (0962) 868020

Riverside
17 Page Street
London SW1P 4NB
Tel: (071) 828 9811
Contact Tel: (081) 846 6388

Wymott
Moss Lane
Ulnes Walton
Leyland
Preston
Lancashire PR5 3LW
Tel: (0772) 421461

Chorley & South Ribble District Offices
Chorley & District General Hospital
Preston Road
Chorley PR7 1PP
Tel: (0257) 261222
Contact Tel: (0257) 245325

The following prisons are due to open between 1992 and 1994. There are no addresses or telephone numbers available at present. When operational, the inquiries section at Cleland House (Prison Department) will be able to assist you – (071) 217 3000. Alternatively, you could telephone a nearby prison if one exists. Such prisons are shown in brackets below.

Blakenhurst, Worcestershire (Hewell Grange)
Doncaster, Yorkshire
Elmley, Kent (Swaleside)
Highdown, Surrey (Downview)
Holme House, Durham
Lancaster Farms, Lancashire
Wolds, Humberside (Everthorpe)
Woodhill, Buckinghamshire.

Appendix 5

Part 2: Directory of Prisons/YOIs, with corresponding Prison Areas and Regional Health Authorities/ Regional HIV Prevention Co-ordinators

Key to Prison Areas

North East	NE	Kent	KT
Yorkshire	YK	The Chilterns	CL
North West	NW	South Coast	SC
Trans Pennine	TP	London South	LS
Mercia	MC	London North	LN
East Midlands	EM	Wessex	WX
Central	CN	Wales and West	WW
East Anglia	EA		

---

1. Northern

Regional AIDS Co-ordinator
(currently Muriel Robinson)
Benfield Road
Newcastle Upon Tyne NE6 4PY
Tel: (091) 224 6222 x 46145

Prisons	Acklington		NE
	Castington		NE
	Deerbolt	YOI	NE
	Durham		NE
	Frankland		NE
	Haverigg		NW
	Kirklevington Grange	YOI	NE
	Low Newton		NE

Total: 8

2. Yorkshire

Regional Health Promotion Officer
(currently Joan Holmes)
The Queen Building
Park Parade
Harrogate HG1 5AH
Tel: (0423) 500066 x 2178

Prisons: Askham Grange   YK
         Everthorpe   YOI   YK
         Full Sutton   NE
         Hull   YK
         Leeds   TP
         New Hall   YOI and Prison   TP
         Northallerton   YOI   YK
         Rudgate   TP
         Thorp Arch   TP
         Wakefield   TP
         Wetherby   YOI   YK

         Total: 11

3. Trent

Regional AIDS Co-ordinator
(currently Rae Magowan)
Fulwood House
Old Fulwood Road
Sheffield S10 3TH
Tel: (0742) 630300 x 640

Prisons: Ashwell   CN
         Foston Hall   MC
         Gartree   CN
         Glen Parva   YOI   CN
         Hatfield   YOI   YK
         Leicester   CN
         Lincoln   EM
         Lindholme   YK
         Moorland   YOI   YK
         Morton Hall   EM
         North Sea Camp   EM
         Nottingham   EM
         Ranby   EM
         Stocken   EM
         Sudbury   MC
         Whatton   EM

         Total: 16

4. East Anglia

Regional HIV Co-ordinator
(currently Dr Mike Rowland)
Union Lane
Chesterton
Cambridge CB4 1RF
Tel: (0223) 61212 x 200

Prisons: Blundeston   EA
         Highpoint   EA
         Hollesley Bay   YOI   EA
         Littlehey   LN
         Norwich   EA
         Wayland   EA
         Whitemore   LN

         Total: 7

5. North West Thames

Regional HIV Co-ordinator
(currently Greg Lucas)
HIV Project
82–86 Seymour Place
London W1H 5DB
Tel: (071) 724 7443

Prisons:		
Bedford	LN
Feltham YOI	LS
The Mount	CL
Wormwood Scrubs	LN

Total: 4

6. North East Thames

Regional HIV Co-ordinator
(currently Rita O'Brien)
40 Eastbourne Terrace
London W2 3QR
Tel: (071) 262 8011 x 2255

Prisons:		
Bullwood Hall YOI and Prison	EA
Chelmsford	EA
Holloway	LN
Pentonville	LN

Total: 4

7. South East Thames

Regional HIV Co-ordinator
(currently Wendy Moreton)
Oak Lodge
David Solomon's House
Broomhill Road
Southborough
Kent TN3 0TG
Tel: (0892) 515152 x 3093

Prisons:		
Aldington	KT
Belmarsh	LS
Blantyre House	KT
Brixton	LS
Canterbury	KT
Cookham Wood	EA
Dover YOI	KT
East Sutton Park YOI and Prison	KT
Lewes	SC
Maidstone	KT
Northeye	SC
Rochester YOI	EA
Standford Hill	KT
Swaleside	KT

Total: 14

8. South West Thames

Regional HIV Services Manager
(currently Martin Weaver)
40 Eastbourne Terrace
London W2 3QR
Tel: (071) 262 8011 x 4091

Prisons:		
Coldingley	CL
Downview	SC
Ford	SC
Latchmere House	LS
Send	SC
Wandsworth	LS

Total: 6

9. Wessex

Regional HIV Co-ordinator
(currently Nicola Woodward)
Highcroft Cottage
Romsey Road
Winchester SO22 5DH
Tel: (0962) 63511 x 376

Prisons:		
Albany		LS
Camp Hill		LS
Parkhurst		LS
Dorchester		WX
Erlestoke House		WW
Guys Marsh	YOI	WX
Haslar	YOI	SC
Kingston		SC
Portland	YOI	WX
The Verne		WX
Winchester		SC

Total: 11

10. Oxford

Regional HIV Co-ordinator
(currently Jonathan Glasson)
Old Road
Headington
Oxford OX3 7LF
Tel: (0865) 226736

Prisons:		
Aylesbury	YOI	CL
Bullingdon		CL
Finnamore Wood	YOI	CL
Grendon		LN
Spring Hill		LN
Huntercombe	YOI	CL
Oxford		CL
Reading		CL
Wellingborough		LN

Total: 9

11. **South Western**

Regional HIV Co-ordinator
(currently Dr Mike Owen)
Dean Clark House
Southernhay East
Exeter EX1 1PQ
Tel: (0392) 406186

Prisons:	Bristol		WW
	Channings Wood		WX
	Dartmoor		WX
	Eastwood Park	YOI	WW
	Exeter		WX
	Gloucester		WW
	Leyhill		WW
	Pucklechurch		WW
	Shepton Mallet		WX

Total: 9

12. **West Midlands**

Regional HIV Co-ordinator
(currently Tom Matthews)
Arthur Thomson House
146 Hagley Road
Birmingham B16 9PA
Tel: (021) 456 1444

Prisons:	Birmingham		CN
	Brinsford	YOI	CN
	Brockhill		MC
	Drake Hall	YOI	
	and Prison		MC
	Featherstone		CN
	Hewell Grange	YOI	MC
	Long Lartin		CN
	Onley	YOI	CL
	Shrewsbury		MC
	Stafford		CN
	Stoke Heath	YOI	MC
	Swinfen Hall	YOI	MC
	Werrington	YOI	MC

Total: 13

13. **Mersey**

Regional HIV Co-ordinator
(currently Howard Seymour)
Hamilton House
24 Pall Mall
Liverpool L3 6AL
Tel: (051) 236 4620 x 2040

Prisons:	Liverpool	TP
	Risley	TP

Styal YOI and Prison		TP
Thorn Cross YOI		NW

Total: 4

14. North Western

Regional HIV Prevention Co-ordinator
(currently Krista Lewis)
Gateway House
Piccadilly South
Manchester M60 7LP
Tel: (061) 237 2610

Prisons:	Garth	NW
	Hindley	NW
	Kirkham	NW
	Lancaster	NW
	Manchester	TP
	Preston	NW
	Wymott	NW

Total: 7

15. Wales

For Cardiff
District Health Care Co-ordinator
(currently Clive Rees)
HIV Co-ordination Centre
Abten House
Wendal Road
Roath
Cardiff CF4 3QX
Tel: (0222) 522011

For Swansea
HIV Co-ordinator
(currently John Duff)
West Glamorgan Social Services
County Hall
Oystermouth Road
Swansea SA1 3SN
Tel: (0792) 471282

For Prescoed and Usk
HIV/AIDS Education and Advice Officer
(currently Gesine Thomas)
Health Promotion Centre
Saint Cadock's Hospital Grounds
Lodge Road
Caerleon
Gwent NP6 1XS
Tel: (0633) 430300

Prisons:	Cardiff		WW
	Prescoed	YOI	WW
	Swansea		WW
	Usk		WW

Total: 4

Appendix 6

Useful Organisations

National AIDS and HIV Organisations

Black HIV/AIDS Network
111 Devonport Road
London W12 8PB
Tel: (081) 742 9223

Provides services to Asian, African and Caribbean people affected by HIV. These include counselling, home care and support. Education and training courses also offered to statutory and voluntary organisations.

Body Positive
National Office
51b Philbeach Gardens
Earl's Court
London SW5 9EB
Telephone Helpline: (071) 373 9124 (Daily 7pm – 10pm)
Admin: (071) 835 1045 (office hours)

Body Positive offers a wide and developing range of services and self-help for people who are HIV antibody positive. The Body Positive Prisoners' Support Group will write to prisoners who feel they would benefit from support.

Prisoners' Support Group:
Address as above. The name of the organisation can be omitted for reasons of confidentiality.

Mainliners
Mainliners Ltd
PO Box 125
London SW9 8EF
Helpline (071) 737 3141 (office hours)

Mainliners is an agency which works for and with drug users affected by HIV.

National AIDS Helpline
A 24-hour national phone line offering advice, information and referral on any aspect of HIV and AIDS for anyone. The call is free.
Helpline: (0800) 567 123 (24 hours)

The helpline is staffed by people who speak:
• Bengali, Gujarati, Hindi, Punjabi and Urdu on Wednesdays 6pm–10pm on (0800) 282 445

- Chinese (Cantonese) on Tuesdays, 6pm–10pm on (0800) 282 446
- Arabic on Wednesdays, 6pm–10pm on (0800) 282 447

A 24-hour recorded message in each language is available on the above numbers outside these times.

For people who are deaf or hard of hearing:
Minicom (0800) 521 361 Daily 10am–10pm

A range of leaflets on HIV and AIDS is available from: Leaflet line:
(0800) 555 777.

Positively Women
5 Sebastian Street
London EC1V 0HE
Tel: (071) 490 5515

Provides counselling and support services for women with HIV or AIDS. They also produce a range of leaflets.

Scottish AIDS Monitor
National office in Edinburgh
PO Box 48
Edinburgh EH1 3SA
Tel: (031) 557 3885

The national HIV and AIDS organisation for Scotland. Its many services include a buddy network, which can include prisoners in certain instances. They also provide training and education for staff and prisoners.

Terrence Higgins Trust (THT)
52–54 Grays Inn Road
London WC1X 9JU
Helpline: (071) 242 1010 3pm–10pm every day.
Information about other services: (071) 831 0330 10am–5pm.

THT provides a range of services for anyone affected by HIV or AIDS. These include a range of leaflets (including *HIV and AIDS: a Booklet for Prisoners*, 1991), support groups, advice and buddying. They employ a prison liaison officer.

Drug Services

There are a range of services available for drug users locally and throughout the country. An important source of local help for the prevention of HIV among injecting drug users are needle and syringe exchanges. Often these services also offer a range of information, advice, counselling, support and referral to drug users, their friends and relatives.

Other types of services offered to drug users are residential rehabilitation, self-help groups, prescribing and other medical assistance.

National Drug Agencies

Institute for the Study of Drug Dependence (ISDD)
1 Hatton Place
Hatton Garden
London EC1N 8ND
Tel: (071) 430 1991

ISDD has an extensive research library (open to anyone by appointment) and produces a range of publications on drugs and their effects.

Release
388 Old Street
London ECIV 9LT
Advice: (071) 729 9904
Administration and Publications: (071) 729 5255.

Advice, information, training and referral on legal and drug-related problems.

Scottish Drugs Forum
5 Oswald Street
Glasgow GI 4QR
Tel: (041) 221 1175

Co-ordinating body for people concerned with drug problems throughout Scotland. Produces a list of local drug agencies in Scotland.

Standing Conference on Drug Abuse (SCODA)
1–4 Hatton Place
Hatton Garden
London ECIN 8ND
Tel: (071) 430 2341

National co-ordinating organisation for drug services. It publishes a directory *Drug Problems: Where to Get Help* which lists drug agencies throughout England and Wales.

Freephone Drug Problems
A recorded message which lists a drug service for every county in England and telephone numbers for Northern Ireland, Scotland and Wales. Dial 100 and ask the operator for Freephone Drug Problems.

Organisations Concerned with Prisons

Howard League for Penal Reform
708 Holloway Road
London N19 3NL
Tel: (071) 281 7722

The Howard League campaigns for a more humane criminal justice system. It produces a newsletter, *Criminal Justice*, and an academic journal entitled *The Howard Journal*. Contact the address above for subscription rates and further information.

National Association for the Care and Resettlement of Offenders (NACRO)
169 Clapham Road
London SW9 0PU
Tel: (071) 582 6500
Membership secretary: (071) 582 5100

NACRO provides various services for ex-prisoners and has an extensive publications list about criminal justice which includes prison topics. There are two different types of membership. It is advisable to contact the membership secretary before subscribing to see which type of membership offers the most appropriate information.

Prison Reform Trust (PRT)
59 Caledonian Road
London N1 9BU
Tel: (071) 278 9815

PRT is a national charity which campaigns for better conditions in prisons and the greater use of alternatives to custody. They produce a quarterly newsletter entitled *Prison Report* and a number of publications. Details of the various types of subscription are available from the above address.

Two publications are of specific relevance: the *Prisoners' Information Pack* is an excellent resource for anyone wanting to know more about issues which prisoners are confronted with. It also includes a list of prison addresses and telephone numbers and helpful information for visitors.

HIV, AIDS and Prisons, first edition 1988, updated 1991, was the first publication to focus on this issue.

Prisoners' Advice Service
708 Holloway Road
London N19 3NL
Tel: (071) 281 4815

The Prisoners' Advice Service takes up prisoners' complaints about their treatment in the prison system by offering free advice and assistance on an individual and confidential basis.

Women in Prison
25 Horsell Road
London N5 1XL
Tel: (071) 609 7463

Women in Prison is an ex-prisoner organisation campaigning on the issues of women's imprisonment. Contact from women prisoners about any aspect of imprisonment is welcome. They employ a welfare worker.

Appendix 7

Keeping up to Date

HIV and AIDS

National AIDS Manual
Subscription details from:
NAM Publications
Unit 407, Brixton Enterprise Centre
London SW9 8EJ
Tel: (071) 737 1846

An invaluable resource addressing key HIV and AIDS issues and providing information on services throughout the country. The manual is in three volumes and is regularly updated. There are sections providing information on prisons, the probation service and HIV and AIDS.

AIDS Dialogue
AIDS Dialogue Distribution Section
Health Education Authority
Hamilton House
Mabledon Place
London WC1H 9TX
Tel: (071) 383 3833

A quarterly magazine published by the Health Education Authority. It provides useful articles about health education initiatives, safer sex, drug use, services, training materials, courses and books. It incorporates *AIDS UK* which gives updates on reported HIV and AIDS figures. Available free to professionals. To be put on the mailing list write to the above address.

Department of Health – AIDS Figures
The AIDS Unit
Friars House
157–168 Blackfriars Road
London SE1 8EU

The Department of Health issues monthly press releases about AIDS. To be put on the mailing list write to the above address. Available free.

AIDS Newsletter
Subscription Office
Bureau of Hygiene and Tropical Diseases
Keppel Street
London WC1E 7HT
Tel: (071) 636 9636

A useful publication for keeping up to date with a wide range of developments. It is published 17 times a year and comprises abstracts based mostly on news cuttings. For details of annual subscription rates write to the above address.

HIV News Review
Terrence Higgins Trust
52–54 Grays Inn Road
London WC1X 8JU
Tel: (071) 831 0330

A quarterly update by the Terrence Higgins Trust covering scientific, social and educational aspects of HIV and AIDS. There are varying subscription rates – write or phone for details.

AIDS Matters
National AIDS Trust
Room 1403
Euston Tower
286 Euston Road
London NW1 3DN
Tel: (071) 383 4246

A newsletter published by the National AIDS Trust. It includes easy to read articles on many issues ranging from HIV and AIDS policy to the needs of particular groups. It is distributed free of charge. Write to NAT to be put on the mailing list.

Body Positive Newsletter
Body Positive Centre
51b Philbeach Gardens
London SW5 9EB.
Tel: (071) 835 1045

A fortnightly newsletter which provides information and news on many aspects of HIV and AIDS. It aims to provide information for people with HIV infection or AIDS. It is available free to people who are antibody positive. Organisations and institutions pay an annual subscription.

Mainliners Newsletter
Mainliners
PO Box 125
London SW9 8EF
Tel: (071) 274 4000 x 315

A monthly newsletter aimed at antibody positive people. It focuses on the needs of drug and alcohol users or ex-users and it covers a wide range of issues. It is free to people who are positive and to drug users. For further details write to the above address.

Drugs

SCODA Newsletter
SCODA
1–4 Hatton Place
Hatton Garden
London EC1N 8ND
Tel: (071) 430 2341

This bi-monthly publication addresses the needs and concerns of organisations in the drugs field and includes articles on HIV and AIDS. Subscription details can be obtained by contacting the Administration Team.

Druglink
Druglink Subscriptions
ISDD
1 Hatton Place
London EC1N 8ND
Tel: (071) 430 1991

A bi-monthly magazine for anyone with a professional or occupational interest in drugs and the response to drug misuse in Britain. It is published by the Institute for the Study of Drug Dependence.

Prisons

Prison Report
Prison Reform Trust
59 Caledonian Road
London N1 9BU
Tel: (071) 278 9815

A quarterly newsletter providing up-to-date information on prisons and the criminal justice system. It frequently contains articles and letters from prison staff and prisoners.

Prison Service Journal
HM Prison Leyhill
Wotton-under-Edge
Gloucestershire
GL2 8HL
Tel: (0454) 260681

The *Prison Service Journal* is produced four times a year and includes articles, reviews, letters, reports and interviews on prison issues. There are occasional supplements on specific topics such as HIV and AIDS. For further details contact Gordon Hill at the address above.

Inside Time
New Bridge Association
1 Thorpe Close
Ladbroke Grove
London W10 5YL
Tel: (081) 969 9133

A national newspaper for prisoners available from the above address.

Glossary

Association
A period of recreation when prisoners are allowed to socialise with each other. They can usually choose whether to watch TV, play pool, board games or some other activity if facilities are available and there are sufficient staff to oversee it.

Counselling
This term is used to describe a range of activities in a prison and it is useful to check exactly what is meant each time the term is employed. The variables tend to be: the level of training counsellors have had; the amount of support and supervision they receive; the privacy possible during a counselling session; the presence or absence of a long-term strategy in work with an individual; the extent to which advice is given or a non-directive approach adopted; the level of confidentiality. In this book the term 'counselling' is used to describe the use of particular learned skills to enable an individual to discuss issues raised by HIV and AIDS. This may include pre- and post-test counselling.

Dental dams (latex squares)
Thin sheets of rubber about five inches square originally designed for use in dental surgery, but which can be used as a protective barrier during oral sex. May also be called 'oral shields'.

Dispersal prisons
For prisoners serving long sentences who need to be kept in high security conditions. People are not normally released direct from these prisons, but are transferred to a lower security prison towards the end of their sentence.

Drugs service
An agency from either the voluntary or statutory sector that offers services to drug users. Services provided can be divided into the following: prescribing; needle and syringe exchange; detoxification; self-help; counselling and support and residential rehabilitation. Agencies may offer more than one of these services.

Fresh Start
The name given to revised working arrangements for prison staff which were introduced by the Home Office in 1987. The aim was: to reduce excessive levels of overtime and increase the basic rate of pay; to enhance the job satisfaction of prison staff and improve regimes for prisoners. In practice these arrangements

seem to have been implemented with some difficulty. Dissent continues over staffing levels and this directly affects the facilities available to prisoners.

Governor grade
A member of the prison management team. The different grades in the hierarchy run from five up to one. Prisons vary in the number of governor grade staff they have according to the regime and size.

Harm minimisation
Practical steps that may be taken to reduce the harm associated with drug use.

Harm reduction
This term is a combination of the terms 'harm minimisation' and 'risk reduction.'

High-risk behaviour
A specific form of behaviour that exposes the individual or others to the risk of infection with HIV.

HIV antibody positive
A blood test result showing that a person has been infected with HIV and has developed antibodies to it.

Homophobia
Prejudice against people who are gay, lesbian or bisexual.

Hospital officer
A prison officer who may have trained as a nurse within the NHS or has attended a course organised by the Prison Medical Service.

Induction courses
Organised by prison staff to help new prisoners settle in to prison life. They vary in length, scope and content. Not all prisons run induction courses.

Local prison
For people either on remand awaiting trial, convicted awaiting sentence, or serving short sentences. They also contain prisoners serving the first part of a longer sentence, who are waiting to be given a security category and allocated to another prison.

Needle and syringe exchange scheme
A type of drug agency where injecting drug users can exchange used needles and syringes for new ones. A range of other services may also be offered such as counselling, advice, referral, free condoms and information on safer drug use and safer sex.

Normal location
Where prisoners normally live, on a wing or a unit, unless segregated or separated in another part of the prison such as the hospital.

Open prisons
These have no physical barrier to prevent prisoners from escaping and therefore are for people deemed to be a low security risk (category D).

Personal officer
A prison officer allocated to take a particular interest in a prisoner and to attend to his or her basic welfare needs.

Pre-release courses
Courses usually run by specially trained staff to help prisoners prepare for their release into the community. They vary in length, scope and content. Not all prisons offer pre-release courses and places on them are often limited.

POA – Prison Officers Association
The trade union which represents uniformed grade officers.

Prison Medical Service
A service within the Prison Department independent of the National Health Service. Some doctors are employed full-time, other doctors visit as required and are paid accordingly.

Risk reduction
Practical measures taken to reduce the risk of people being exposed to HIV infection through either drug use or sexual behaviour.

Safer drug use
Ways of using drugs that reduce the risk of transmission of HIV and hepatitis B. Safer drug use therefore does not necessarily mean giving up drugs.

Safer sex
Ways of having sex that reduce the risk of HIV infection, other sexually transmitted diseases and pregnancy.

Security categories for prisoners
Prisoners are categorised as follows:
A. Prisoners whose escape would be highly dangerous to the public or to the security of the state.
B. Prisoners for whom the highest conditions of security are not necessary but for whom escape must be made very difficult.
C. Prisoners who cannot be trusted in open conditions but who do not have the ability or resources to make a determined escape attempt.
D. Those who can reasonably be trusted in open conditions.

Some prisons contain more than one category of prisoner, but the security category of the prison determines the regime which operates there. This means, for example, that a category C prisoner at a category B prison will not receive category C home leave entitlements.

Sharps box
A container used to dispose safely of used needles and syringes.

Slopping out
Prisoners who do not have access to sanitation overnight or when locked up have to use a pot. The contents are emptied by the prisoners in the toilet area when they are unlocked. The Home Secretary has pledged to end this unpleasant situation by the end of 1994.

Training officer
A senior or principal officer who is responsible for organising the staff training programme and managing any training facilities within the prison.

Voluntary organisation
A non-profit making organisation. The term voluntary organisation does not mean that it is staffed by volunteers.

Works
A term used to describe some of the equipment used for injecting drugs, including needle, syringe and spoon.

YOI – Young Offender Institution
Formerly called borstals, youth custody and detention centres. Establishments for 14–21-year-old males and 15–21-year-old females. They may have either open or closed conditions.

Bibliography

Advisory Council on the Misuse of Drugs (1988) *AIDS and Drug Misuse*, Part 1, HMSO, London.

Aggleton, P., Homans, H., Mojsa, J., Watson, S. and Watney, S. (1988) *Learning About AIDS*, Churchill Livingstone, Edinburgh.

Aggleton, P., Homans, H., Mojsa, J., Watson, S. and Watney, S. (1989) *AIDS: Scientific and Social Issues* (included in *Learning About AIDS* but available separately), Churchill Livingstone, Edinburgh.

AIDS Inside (1987) Directorate of the Prison Medical Service, Home Office, London.

Aids Inside and Out (1989) Directorate of the Prison Medical Service, Home Office, London.

Blackburn, D. (1991) *HIV/AIDS Awareness Training for Women in Prison*. Unpublished dissertation for Certificate in Multi-disciplinary Studies of Drug Misuse, Ruskin College, University of Oxford.

Caring for Drug Users: a Multi-disciplinary Resource for People Working with Prisoners (1991) Directorate of the Prison Medical Service, Home Office, London.

Chirimuuta, Richard and Rosalind (1989) *AIDS, Africa and Racism*, Free Association Books, London.

Clark, M. (1990) 'The prison officer as an AIDS trainer and counsellor', *Prison Service Journal*, No. 78, Spring, HM Prison Leyhill, Wotton-under-Edge.

Custody, Care and Justice: the Way Ahead for the Prison Service in England and Wales (1991) Cm 1647, HMSO, London.

Greenwood, Dr J. (1991), speaking at AIDS and Drugs conference organised by the Alcohol Research Group, University of Edinburgh.

HIV and AIDS: a Multi-disciplinary Approach in the Prison Environment (1991) Directorate of the Prison Medical Service, Home Office, London.

HIV Project Information File (1990) North West Thames Regional Health Authority.

Lockley, P. and Williams, M. (1989) *HIV/AIDS Counselling: Trainer's Pack,* Scottish Health Education Group, Edinburgh (now Health Education Board for Scotland).

Mandel, S. (1988) *Effective Presentation Skills*, Kogan Page, London.

Miller, D. and Curran, L. (1991) *The Second Sentence: the Experience and Needs of Prisoners with HIV in HM Prison System, England and Wales*, HM Prison Service.

Moody, D., Aggleton, P. Kapila, M., Pye, M. and Young, A. (1991) *Monitoring and Evaluating Local HIV/AIDS Health Promotion: a Review of Theory and Practice*, HIV, AIDS and Sexual Health Programme, Paper 11, Health Education Authority.

NACRO (1987) *Working with Prisons*, NACRO, London.

Richardson, D. (1990) *Safer Sex: the Guide for Women Today*, Pandora, London.

Smack in the Eye, North West Regional Drug Training Unit, Manchester.

Statement from the Consultation on Prevention and Control of AIDS in Prisons (1987) World Health Organisation, Global Programme on AIDS, Geneva.

Terrence Higgins Trust (1991) *HIV and AIDS: a Booklet for Prisoners*, Terrence Higgins Trust, London.

Turnbull, P., Dolan, K. and Stimson, G. (1991) *Prisons, HIV and AIDS: Risks and Experiences in Custodial Care*, AVERT, London.

User's Guide to Safer Drug Use (1989) Community Drug Project, London.

Woolf, Lord Justice and Tumim, Judge Stephen (1991) *Prison Disturbances April 1990: Report of an Inquiry*, [The Woolf Report], Cm 1456, HMSO, London.

Index

Advisory Council on the Misuse of Drugs
   (ACMD)   11, 165
AIDS: Scientific and Social Issues (Aggleton *et al*,
   1989)   40, 76, 165
AIDS Advisory Committee   6–8
AIDS, Africa and Racism (Chirimuuta &
   Chirimuuta, 1989)   40, 165
AIDS Dialogue   157
AIDS and Drug Misuse (ACMD report)   11, 165
AIDS education packages *see* training packages
AIDS Inside and Out (video)   7, 23, 66–7
   tutor's manual   127
   women's needs and   89
AIDS Inside (video)   6, 165
AIDS Matters   77, 158
AIDS Newsletter   157–8
AIDS Working with Young People (Aggleton *et al*,
   1990)   127
alcohol
   role in HIV transmission   59
   Suffolk Community Alcohol Service   88
   Woolf Report on   119–22
Alcoholics Anonymous   87, 120
alternative therapies   89
Angel Project,   89
Askham Grange Prison   96
attitude statement exercise   27, 50–1; prejudice

bail hostels   11
Belmarsh Prison   13, 19
Black HIV/AIDS Network   153
bleach, to clean injecting equipment   4, 59, 86
Body Positive   6, 92, 153
   Body Positive Newsletter   158
   Body Positive North East   96
Brinsford Young Offenders Institution   90
Bristol Prison   13
   HIV education initiatives   82–4
   Woolf Report on   124
Brook Advisory Service   81
Bullwood Hall Young Offenders Institution   12

cannabis users   121
Caring for Drug Users   97, 165
Central London Action on Street Health
   (CLASH)   88, 89
Community Drug Project (London)   77
community prisons   97
community-based agencies   97–110, 122
condoms
   Bristol Prison policy   83

Hollesley Bay policy   88
Holloway Prison policy   90
   safer sex exercise   61–3
   unavailable in prisons   4
confidentiality issues   5
   in prisons   45, 101–2
   on training course   45
   Woolf Report on   125, 126
Cookham Wood Prison   12
counselling   161
   at Bristol Prison   83–4
   at Feltham   17
   at Hollesley Bay   87
   at Holloway Prison   89–90
   at Saughton Prison   82
   groupwork confidentiality problems   101–2
   HIV/AIDS Counselling: Trainer's Pack   127, 165
   pre- and post-HIV testing   8, 89
   shortage of counsellors   8
   upsetting sessions   101
   Woolf Report on   124
Curran, Len   6
Custody Care and Justice (White Paper)   97, 165

deaths in prisons
   from AIDS-related diseases   3
   suicides   3
dental dams   61, 62, 161
Directorate of Prison Medical Service (DPMS)
   approves HIV/AIDS project   12
   HIV training initiatives   6–8
   HIV/AIDS management policy   122–3
   Prison Brokerage Scheme and   95
   VIR review by   6
Done, Peter   95
Dorchester Prison   84
Drake Hall Young Offenders Institution   90,
   91, 92
dress code
   for courses   31
   when visiting prisons   103
Drug Training, HIV and AIDS in the 1990s   127
drug use   3, 4
   amongst young offenders   87
   community-based drug agencies   97, 154–5
   drug services/agencies   154–5
   drug use exercise   58–60
   in Edinburgh   80, 81
   Grendon Prison policy   86
   Holloway Prison policy   90
   newsletters/magazines   158–9

prison situation exercise   56
Safer Drug Use   166
unidentified   11
User's Guide to Safer Drug Use   77
Woolf Report on   119–22
Druglink   159
Durham prisons   95–6

Effective Presentation Skills (Mandel, 1988)   77
employment issues, prisoner unemployment   3
evaluation, of HIV/AIDS training course   31–3

Featherstone Prison   90
Feltham Young Offenders Institution   12,
    15–17
Fresh Start   161–2

Gamblers Anonymous   120
Gartree Prison   93
Glen Parva Young Offenders Institution   93
Gloucester Prison   84
governor (prison), initial contact to   21–2, 99
Grendon Prison   85–6, 122
groupwork
    confidentiality issues   101–2
    working techniques   115–18
Gunn, Professor   119–22

handouts
    guide to using   76–7
    training methods   115–18
Health Education Authority   11
Health Education Board for Scotland   82
Healthy Options Team   88
*HIV and AIDS: A Training Pack for Young
    People*   127
HIV and AIDS: a Booklet for Prisoners   8, 154
HIV, AIDS and Prisons   156
HIV education packages *see* training packages
HIV News Review   158
HIV testing   5
    Grendon policy on   86
    limited validity of negative result   5
    pre- and post-test counselling   8, 89
    prison situation exercise   55–7
    Woolf Report on   122–3
HIV-positive prisoners
    cumulative totals   4
    disclosure   56, 123
    prejudice against   11, 124, 125
    prison situation exercise   55–7
    The Second Sentence (Miller & Curran,
        1991)   166
    VIR and   4–5, 122–6
HIV/AIDS Counselling: Trainer's Pack   127
Holland, drug-free prison units   121
Hollesley Bay Young Offenders
    Institution   86–8

Holloway Prison   12
    drug withdrawal policy   90, 122
    HIV/AIDS education policy   88–90
homophobia   63, 162
Howard League for Penal Reform   155

injecting drug users *see* drug use
Inside Time   159
Institute for the Study of Drug Dependence
    (ISDD)   154

KI unit (Wandsworth Prison)   5
    Woolf report on   123–4, 125

latex squares   61, 62, 161
Learning About AIDS (education pack)   16, 127,
    165
Leeds Prison   95
Leicestershire HIV/AIDS and Drugs Prison
    Project   93–4
Lifeline Project (Manchester)   77, 86, 120–1

McKenzie, Pat   90–3
Mainliners   89, 153
    newsletter   86, 158
Manchester Prison   95, 96
Marlow, Geoff   16
Mentally disordered prisoners (Gunn
    Report)   119–22
Mojsa, Jan   16, 77, 115–18
myths *see* prejudice

NACRO   79, 94, 96, 155
    Working with Prisons   166
name game exercise   41
NAPO   121, 125
Narcotics Anonymous   87
National AIDS Helpline   153–4
National AIDS Manual   105, 157
National AIDS and Prisons Consortium
    Project   94, 125
National AIDS and Prisons Forum   125
National AIDS Trust   94, 125, 158
National Association for the Care and
    Resettlement of Offenders *see* NACRO
National Association of Probation
    Officers   121, 125
needle exchange schemes   59, 162
Netherlands, drug-free prison units   121

oral sex, protection during   61, 62, 161
oral shields   61, 62, 161
overcrowding   3
Parole Release Scheme   16–17, 18, 94, 96
Pentonville Prison   12, 17–18
Portland Prison   84

Positively Women   89, 154
pre-release courses
    at Bristol Prison   83
    at Hollesley Bay   88
prejudice
    against HIV-positive prisoners   11, 124, 125
    attitude statement exercise   27, 50–1
    dealing with difficult issues   39–40
    facts *versus* myths exercise   48–9
    homophobic attitudes   63, 162
    moral dilemmas role play   52–4
    prison situation exercise   55–7
Prison Brokerage Scheme   94–6
prison disturbances   3
Prison Medical Service *see* Directorate of Prison
    Medical Service
Prison Reform Trust   102, 104, 155–6
Prison Report   159
Prison Service Journal   77, 159
Prisoners Advice and Legal Service   104, 156
Prisoners' Information Pack   102, 156
prisons
    directory of   129–52
    newsletters/journals   159
    organisations concerned with   155–6
    working with community agencies   97–110
    working with outsiders   106–8
    working with prisoners   101–5, 109
    see also individual institutions
probation hostels   11

questionnaires
    for course evaluation   31–3, 34
    training needs analyses   113–14

reception into prison   122–3
    at Grendon Prison   85
    drug use denied   11
    HIV status denied   124
Release   155
riots   3
Robertson, Di   94–6

Safer Drug Use   166
safer sex   163
Safer Sex: the Guide for Women Today
    (Richardson, 1990)   62, 166
    Saughton Prison initiative   81–2
    The A–Z of safer sex (poster)   77
    training exercise   61–3
Samaritans   89
sanitation in prisons   3, 164
Saughton Prison   13
    HIV/AIDS education initiatives   80–2
    Woolf Report on   124
SCODA   59, 105, 155
    newsletter   158–9
Scottish AIDS Monitor   154

Scottish Drugs Forum   155
Scottish Health Education Group   82
Scottish prison system   2
    Saughton Prison   13, 80–2, 124
sexual activity in prisons   4
slopping out   164
Smack in the Eye   86, 166
Spring Hill Prison   86
staff (prison)
    counselling training   8
    education packages designed by   23, 25–6,
        65–7
    training needs analyses   113–14
    training of uniformed staff only   14
Stafford Prison   90, 91
Standing Conference on Drug Abuse
    (SCODA)   59, 105, 155
    newsletter   158–9
statistics
    AIDS-related deaths in prisons   3
    Department of Health – AIDS Figures   157
    people with AIDS in UK   76
    prison suicides   3
substance abuse *see* drug use
Suffolk Community Alcohol Service   88
suicides in prison, in 1990   3
Swinfen Hall Young Offenders Institution   90
syringe/needle exchange schemes   59, 162

teachers *see* training exercises
Terrence Higgins Trust   154
    AIDS Advisory Committee and   6
    HIV and AIDS booklet   8, 154
    HIV News Review   158
    Holloway Prison involvement   89
    National AIDS and Prisons Consortium
        Project and   94
training exercises   37–77
    attitude statement   50–1
    devising an education package   65–7
    difficult questions carousel   68–70
    drug use   58–60
    expectations   46–7
    facts *versus* myths   48–9
    ground rules   44–5
    groupwork methods   115–18
    handouts, guide to using   76–7
    moral dilemmas role play   52–4
    name game   41
    opening/closing session   42–3, 115
    presentation practice   72–3
    prison situations   55–7
    safer sex   61–3
    training methods discussion   64
    training methods handout   115–18
    training resource list   127
training needs analyses   113–14

training packages   7–8
    at Bristol Prison   82–4
    at Grendon Prison   85–6
    at Hollesley Bay   86–8
    at Holloway Prison   88–90
    at Saughton Prison   80–2
    designed by staff   23, 25–6, 65–7
    in Leicestershire prisons   93–4
    organising training of staff   25–35
    Prison Brokerage Scheme   94–6
    in Staffordshire prisons   90–3
    training exercises   37–77
Tumin, Judge Stephen *see* Woolf Report

unemployment (prisoner)   3
updates on HIV/AIDS   34

videos
    AIDS Inside   6
    AIDS Inside and Out   7, 23, 66–7, 127, 89
VIR *see* Viral Infectivity Restrictions
Viral Infectivity Restrictions (VIR)
    applied to HIV   4–6
    not adopted in Scotland   80
    not used at Grendon   85
    Stafford Prison policy   91
    Woolf Report on   6, 123–6

Wandsworth Prison (KI unit)   5
    Woolf Report on   123–4, 125
Werrington Young Offenders Institution   90
Whitlock, Sue   93–4

Winchester Prison   84
Women in Prison (London)   156
women prisoners   13
    Bulwood Hall   12
    Drake Hall   90, 91, 92
    HIV/AIDS Awareness Training (Blackburn,
        1981)   165
    Holloway Prison   12, 88–90
Wool, Dr Rosemary   88
Woolf Report   166
    on community prisons   97
    on community-based agencies   97
    extracts from   119–26
    on management of drug abusers   119–22
    on management of HIV/AIDS   122–6
    on prison staff development   14
    VIR review recommended by   6, 125
Working with Uncertainty (Dixon & Gordon,
        1988)   127
World Health Organisation, statement on AIDS
    in prisons   77

Young Offender Institutions   15, 164
    Brinsford   90
    directory of   129–52
    Drake Hall   90, 91, 92
    Feltham   12, 15–17
    Glen Parva   93
    Hollesley Bay   86–8
    Swinfen Hall   90
    Werrington   90